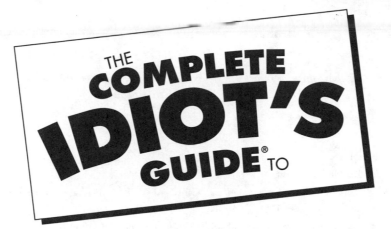

THE COMPLETE IDIOT'S GUIDE® TO

Core Conditioning

Illustrated

by *Patrick S. Hagerman, Ed.D.*

ALPHA

A member of Penguin Group (USA) Inc.

This book is dedicated to all those unsung muscles in your body that have never been given the attention they deserve. Here's to all the little guys that hold you up.

ALPHA BOOKS

Published by the Penguin Group

Penguin Group (USA) Inc., 375 Hudson Street, New York, New York 10014, U.S.A.

Penguin Group (Canada), 10 Alcorn Avenue, Toronto, Ontario, Canada M4V 3B2 (a division of Pearson Penguin Canada Inc.)

Penguin Books Ltd., 80 Strand, London WC2R 0RL, England

Penguin Ireland, 25 St Stephen's Green, Dublin 2, Ireland (a division of Penguin Books Ltd.)

Penguin Group (Australia), 250 Camberwell Road, Camberwell, Victoria 3124, Australia (a division of Pearson Australia Group Pty. Ltd.)

Penguin Books India Pvt. Ltd., 11 Community Centre, Panchsheel Park, New Delhi—110 017, India

Penguin Group (NZ), cnr Airborne and Rosedale Roads, Albany, Auckland 1310, New Zealand (a division of Pearson New Zealand Ltd.)

Penguin Books (South Africa) (Pty.) Ltd., 24 Sturdee Avenue, Rosebank, Johannesburg 2196, South Africa

Penguin Books Ltd., Registered Offices: 80 Strand, London WC2R 0RL, England

International Standard Book Number: 1-59257-456-4
Library of Congress Catalog Card Number: 2005935923

08 07 06   8 7 6 5 4 3 2 1

Interpretation of the printing code: The rightmost number of the first series of numbers is the year of the book's printing; the rightmost number of the second series of numbers is the number of the book's printing. For example, a printing code of 06-1 shows that the first printing occurred in 2006.

Printed in the United States of America

Note: This publication contains the opinions and ideas of its author. It is intended to provide helpful and informative material on the subject matter covered. It is sold with the understanding that the author and publisher are not engaged in rendering professional services in the book. If the reader requires personal assistance or advice, a competent professional should be consulted.

The author and publisher specifically disclaim any responsibility for any liability, loss, or risk, personal or otherwise, which is incurred as a consequence, directly or indirectly, of the use and application of any of the contents of this book.

Most Alpha books are available at special quantity discounts for bulk purchases for sales promotions, premiums, fund-raising, or educational use. Special books, or book excerpts, can also be created to fit specific needs.

For details, write: Special Markets, Alpha Books, 375 Hudson Street, New York, NY 10014.

Publisher: *Marie Butler-Knight*
Editorial Director/Acquiring Editor: *Mike Sanders*
Senior Managing Editor: *Jennifer Bowles*
Development Editor: *Lynn Northrup*
Senior Production Editor: *Billy Fields*
Copy Editor: *Krista Hansing*

Cartoonist: *Shannon Wheeler*
Book Designer: *Trina Wurst*
Cover Designer: *Bill Thomas*
Indexer: *Tonya Heard*
Layout: *Becky Harmon*
Proofreading: *Donna Martin*

Contents at a Glance

Contents

Foreword

Core training is the biggest training phenomenon to come down the pike in the last decade. Core is everywhere and you cannot escape it. I spoke on core training at a national conference a year ago and core was a consistent theme everywhere I turned. There were many vendors with the word "core" for the name of their company, or "core" as the name of a piece of equipment, or "core" on some type of book or manual. It's huge.

After speaking to various groups, working with fitness buffs, and training personal trainers on the core, I have come to see that there is a lot of confusion about the core. An owner of a running store wanted me to come speak on the core and I said, "Great, I have a DVD called *3D Abs* and my passion is to train and educate people on this." She replied, "We don't want ab training, we want core training." I wanted to tell her that it's the same thing, but I did not want to embarrass her. Obviously this person was only partially informed. There is widespread research and training techniques concerning the core from various camps and it can be daunting to sort through it without a guide. Dr. Hagerman is the guide.

Dr. Hagerman brings clarity to the topic without being too "researchy" or too superficial. He covers all the details as well as gives the big picture. He cuts through the myths regarding core training and addresses what's relevant for the fitness person in the trenches.

Dr. Hagerman is not only a professor who is well-versed in teaching and research, he also works out and works out hard. He knows what's relevant from experience. This is a step-by-step system that works. Dr. Hagerman states, "It takes more than 3 minutes a day to get the results you are after. A good core workout should last about 30 minutes." After designing a 3D workout, teaching it, and working it, I couldn't agree more. This is no fluff. Whether you are a beginner or more advanced, *The Complete Idiot's Guide to Core Conditioning Illustrated* gives you the exercises necessary to get strong and enhance definition.

Not only does Dr. Hagerman cover the tried-and-true basic abdominal exercises, he also presents the new trendy ones as well as creating advanced ones I have never seen before. Do you ever get tired of doing just ONE abdominal exercise? Do crunches day after day bore you? This stuff is actually fun. You can do an exercise that challenges your balance and your agility, and your core gets worked out in the process. It's multi-system.

With over 100 exercises, you have plenty to choose from. After teaching courses on the core, I have come to realize how important it is to emphasize proper form and technique. Participants display all kinds of compensations that inhibit them from loading the core and getting the most out of a particular exercise. The pictures and explanations in this book are very thorough and alleviate any confusion on the reader's behalf. When I read it I realized I had a preconceived idea about what I "thought" it would cover. Well, I was pleasantly surprised in that it is a great resource for working out in general. It covers everything from staying motivated to knowing if an exercise will hurt your back. *The Complete Idiot's Guide to Core Conditioning Illustrated* is a great reference tool and somewhat of a "core bible."

—Michael Griffith, PT, CSCS

A physical therapist with physique in mind, Michael's expertise and focus is performance analysis of athletes with an emphasis on core function and training. He has written articles for journals and fitness magazines. He has hosted seminars and discussions across the country regarding core training.

Introduction

Today fitness is one of the largest industries in the world. Every bookstore has shelves lined with all types of exercise programs, late-night infomercials try to sell the latest and greatest gadget that will transform your body by the next morning, and plenty of diets promise to burn fat and build muscles like you wouldn't believe. Well, *I* don't believe. Fitness is a constant topic everywhere you look, but at the same time, the fitness level of our population is going down.

It's time something changed. For too long, exercise programs have focused on what you look like on the outside, ignoring all the muscles deeper within your body that form the foundation of your fitness. You may look great on the outside, but if your base isn't solid, that look can come tumbling down at any moment. That's why core conditioning is so important. Core training starts on the inside, helping you build a firm foundation for other exercise programs to grow from. It takes time, but the results you get will stay with you forever. If you start strong, you'll end up strong—it's that simple.

This book provides all the tools you need to get started on building a solid core-conditioning program. You'll come away with a better grasp of what is happening inside your body every time you move, what muscles are contributing to your success, and how to train them the right way every time. By following the advice in this book, you'll quickly be on your way to a fitter, stronger, more healthy body that's the envy of everyone you know.

How to Use This Book

The book is separated into three parts, each of which covers an essential component of core conditioning:

Part 1, "Getting to the Center of Your Body," explains the basics of core conditioning, including how it differs from other exercise programs, along with some basic anatomy and science to support it. It also provides you with the tools to develop your own core-conditioning program so you know exactly what you need to do during every workout.

Part 2, "Targeting Movements, Not Muscles," is the heart of your core-conditioning program. In these chapters, you will find all the information you need to maximize your core-conditioning workout. This information includes step-by-step instructions and photographs of a wide range of exercises to train every muscle in your core in every possible direction. Chapters are divided by the type of resistance used and the difficulty level of the exercises, and are even presented in a simple-to-complex format so you know exactly what exercise to do next.

Part 3, "Keeping in Touch," covers two more essential elements of core conditioning: cardiovascular exercise and flexibility training. This is not your normal information, either—it's designed to enhance your core-conditioning program with exercises and stretches that focus on those same muscles so the results you get are exactly what you want. With these guides, you will come out of your workouts feeling complete and ready to go. The final chapter will help keep you focused on your goal and moving toward a better body every day.

Extras

Throughout this book, you'll also find sidebars with quick and important pieces of information that summarize some of the text or add information that's important to know. These sidebars include the following:

Getting Defined

In these boxes, you'll find definitions of terms you may not know.

Six-Pack Says

These inspiring quotes from fitness professionals will help keep you motivated.

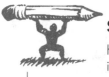

Suck It In

Here you'll find tips for maximizing your training program.

Don't Throw It Out

Check these special cautions to keep you safe.

So read on, start moving, and good luck. The key to success is consistency, form, and commitment. I know you can do it!

Acknowledgments

This book has been a major project over the last few months. Since it is really one of the first core conditioning books, there was a lot of research to be done, which meant a lot of time at the library. I want to thank my wife, Becki, for all her help and support. From cooking lunch during photo shoots, to making sure I stayed in my office and finished that chapter I'd been putting off, she was a great help. I love you.

To my students and friends who agreed to model for pictures (there were some long days in the studio), I appreciate your patience and help. A big thanks goes to Jay Dawes, Jenifer Anderson, Michael Griffith, Sara Fletcher, Nicole Scott, and Aaron Edwards.

Finally, thanks to everyone I called upon to get quotes and answer questions. Sometimes things sound simple in your head but get confusing on paper. I needed help from time to time to make sure it all made sense—and I think we got the job done.

Trademarks

All terms mentioned in this book that are known to be or are suspected of being trademarks or service marks have been appropriately capitalized. Alpha Books and Penguin Group (USA) Inc. cannot attest to the accuracy of this information. Use of a term in this book should not be regarded as affecting the validity of any trademark or service mark.

In This Part

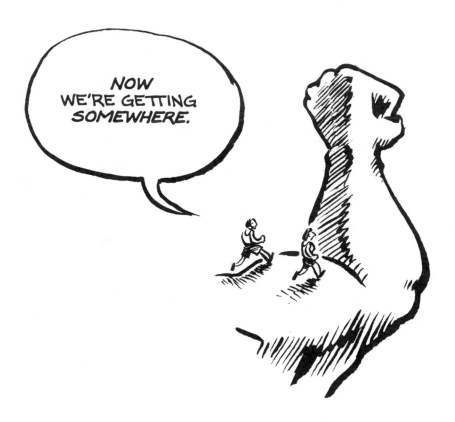

Getting to the Center of Your Body

How to build a solid foundation is the first thing you learn in any engineering class. The same thing should be taught in every exercise program. Without a firm base to build upon, strength and endurance improvements are harder to achieve and even more difficult to keep. Core conditioning is the foundation for all other exercise programs to build upon, so it should be the starting point for your new workout plan.

Part 1 discusses why core conditioning is such an important part of your fitness goals and how it is different from all other types of exercise programs. You will learn the subtle nuances that separate a good conditioning program from an ineffective one. You'll see that there are a whole lot of muscles in your body that you've never even felt before. Finally, Part 1 gives you all the tools you need to build your core-conditioning program from the ground up, including expert recommendations on the number of reps, sets, and exercises to do every day, along with the proper equipment you'll need to get that foundation built.

In This Chapter

- ◆ Finding your core
- ◆ Feeling more than seeing
- ◆ How core conditioning differs from other exercise regimes
- ◆ Training like the pros

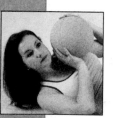
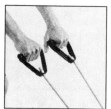
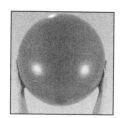
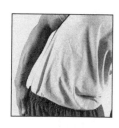
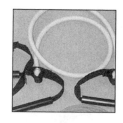
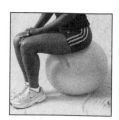

Chapter 1

What Is Core Conditioning?

If you walk up to someone on the street and ask them to point to their core, chances are that person will give you a funny look and say he has no idea where that is. Since you are reading this now, you must have some idea where your core is located and what it does—so that makes my job easier. If you aren't familiar with it, I'll start by telling you that core conditioning is one of the latest breakthroughs in exercise science and is quickly becoming a foundation for all other exercise programs.

Historically, our drive for fitness was fueled by a desire to look and feel good. While there is nothing wrong with that, exercise programs in the past have mainly dealt with the muscles that you can see in the mirror, ignoring the muscles deep within our body that contribute to every move we make. This is where core conditioning comes in.

Where Is Your Core?

Your *core* is basically the trunk of your body—everything except for your arms, legs, and head. Sometimes you may see the core defined as just your abdominal muscles, or your abs and lower back combined. In reality, your core is what allows you to move. It is the part of your body to which everything is attached and from which every movement is controlled. No matter what you are doing—sitting in a chair, pushing a grocery cart down the aisle, playing with your kids, or throwing a softball—your core muscles are involved. After reading this chapter, you'll understand that the muscles you can't see are an important part of a well-rounded fitness program and a style of training that will change the way you move and feel forever.

Getting Defined

The **core** of your body includes everything from your neck to your waist. The muscles of the core help you move and stabilize your arms and legs. Most of them are so deep within the body that you can't actually see them.

Training What You Can't See

If you are asking "Why should I train my core muscles?" you aren't alone. Until recently, core conditioning was a style of training that very few understood and even fewer actually did. It has taken decades of research and understanding how the body moves to decipher how we should train. Although exercise scientists like myself are still looking for even more information, what we do know right now is that you can't isolate a few muscles in your exercise program and expect the other muscles in your body to improve all by themselves.

One of the main principles of exercise states that if you want a muscle to get stronger, you have to make sure you are actually working that muscle. This basically means that if you want your arms to get stronger, you have to train your arms, not your legs. The same goes for every muscle in your body: you get out of it what you put into it. It's still important to train the muscles of your arms and legs, but a whole other group of muscles contributes to your ability to move your arms and legs that you cannot ignore. Core conditioning will enhance the effects of other exercise programs and provide you with more results than you ever imagined!

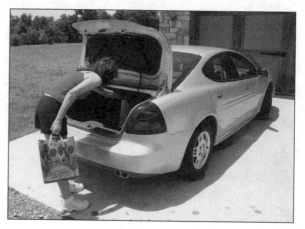

Just getting the groceries out of your trunk requires a stable core so you can bend and lift.

Core conditioning is sometimes referred to as "functional training" because you are working muscles that help you do the things that you do every day—not just muscles that will make you look good in that new swimsuit. You may not ever think about how you unload the dishwasher, climb in and out of your car, or get up off the couch, but you should. Every movement you make is possible because muscles are working. Most of the time, there is more going on in your body than you know about. The "surface" muscles—the ones you can see in the mirror—are mostly responsible for big movements. The "deep" core muscles help stabilize and control the surface muscles so everything works together. One cannot work without the other. In fact, if you listen really closely while you are exercising, you will hear your body singing the chorus of "We are family … I got all these muscles in me."

Core conditioning by itself is only part of a complete exercise program, but it's definitely the part that will improve how you feel throughout the day while you're going about your normal chores. A complete core-conditioning program is going to include strengthening exercises, flexibility exercises, and aerobic work. All three components are covered in this book, so don't skip anything.

Six-Pack Says

Just because you can't see a muscle doesn't mean you don't use it.
—Keith Cinea, Education Department, National Strength and Conditioning Association

Not Your Normal Weight Training

Core conditioning is different from almost every other exercise program you have ever used, and not just because of the exercises involved. Typically, weight-training programs are designed to make you stronger and more able to lift weights that you would never lift in everyday life. When was the last time you needed to actually push 200 pounds off your chest while lying down? Unless you are a professional wrestler, you probably never do this, but it's very common to see people doing heavy bench-press exercises as part of their normal weight-training routines.

Weight training is all about getting stronger. I don't discount the importance of strength, but do you ever think about what muscles are helping your arms and chest perform a bench press? What muscles are stabilizing your arms so that you push up and not out? What muscles are keeping you from dislocating your shoulder? This is what core conditioning is all about—working those muscles that can improve your weight-training workout. It's a whole different style of training because you aren't going to try to make specific muscles stronger; you're trying to make whole groups of muscles stronger and better able to help you in other ways.

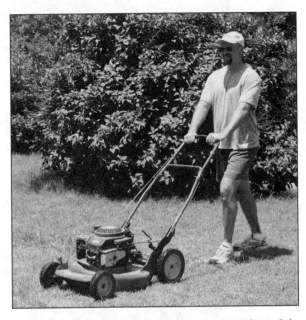

Pushing a lawn mower requires strength and a solid core, and is way more functional than pushing heavy weights.

When you are weight training, you normally use free weights or machines to provide the resistance. In a core-conditioning program, very little resistance is used, and you are never sitting in a machine. Weight training often relies on equipment to stabilize your body while you push or pull on a weight. Core conditioning relies on the other muscles in your body for stabilization while you perform the movement.

Core conditioning and weight training can work together—I actually recommend that you do both. A complete, well-rounded training program has to include weight training and core conditioning because each style of training gives you specific results that neither one can deliver alone. The big difference is that core conditioning is going to improve the way you feel and move rather than increase how much weight you can lift.

Don't Throw It Out

Don't discard your weight-training program for a core-conditioning program. They are meant to work together to help you achieve new levels of fitness.

Different from Body Sculpting

Body sculpting is all about getting a certain look, whether it's big and brawny, cut and defined, or slender and shapely. Core conditioning is unlike body sculpting because you won't really notice any changes on the outside. With core conditioning, it's what you feel that makes the difference, not what you see. Body sculpting is important because it helps you obtain the outward appearance you desire and the healthy body you need. Core conditioning works right along with body sculpting because it works from the inside, providing a solid platform for you to build upon and get even greater results.

Core conditioning can be done just about anywhere. In Chapter 3, I introduce the equipment you can use. With a body-sculpting program, once you reach a certain level, you almost have to have access to a health club or gym because of the equipment you will need to further your program. Advancing your core-conditioning program is simply a matter of changing the exercises to provide more of a challenge; you don't need more and bigger equipment to do it. In fact, in a core-conditioning program, once you reach a certain level of strength and ability, the resistance doesn't increase because you aren't trying to make the muscles bigger or more defined. Your goal is to get your muscles working properly and in coordination with the larger surface muscles that a body-sculpting program concentrates on.

Both programs actually have a few exercises in common. A few of the core muscles are also surface muscles that you would train with a body-sculpting program. For example, the major abdominal muscle that gives you the six-pack look is also a major core muscle that provides a lot of stabilization. The difference is that a core-conditioning program focuses on how the muscle works rather than how it looks, so no getting a six-pack here.

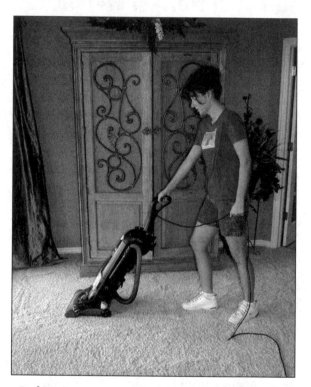

Pushing a vacuum won't give you sculpted abs, but your core abdominals are responsible for all the rotation.

It Looks Like Pilates and Yoga

Looks can be deceiving. Core conditioning may look like some of the same exercises you might do in a Pilates or yoga program, but they don't feel the same. Pilates floor or mat exercises don't require much in the way of equipment, and they actually activate many of the same muscles as a core-conditioning program, but not in the same way. Pilates floor exercises are usually done in slower, more concentrated motions than core conditioning. A core program is often completed faster, with more dynamic movements involving balance, coordination, and power that Pilates doesn't cover. Advanced Pilates requires big, fancy equipment that costs more money than all but the richest people can afford—not so with core conditioning. As I mentioned, advancing a program is as simple as changing the exercises, not the equipment.

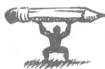

Suck It In _____

Core conditioning, yoga, and Pilates are all different forms of exercise, each with its own style and purpose. The trick is, having a stronger core helps you in more than one way—it even makes you better at yoga and Pilates.

Yoga is different as well. Yoga requires a lot of flexibility to be done right—and that can take years of training (or decades, if you're like me). Yoga postures are done smoothly and slowly, whereas core conditioning often has a hint of power and speed that really gets your body working. The only equipment you use in yoga is your body. Core conditioning trains you to respond to outside resistance while you are moving; yoga can't do that. I agree that flexibility is a part of a complete core-conditioning program, but flexibility is not a main objective or requirement for improving the condition of your core muscles. Furthermore, yoga and Pilates do not incorporate aerobic training, which is an essential element of proper core conditioning.

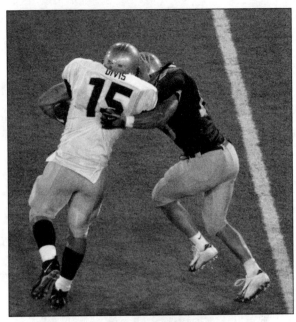

Football players rely on a solid core to keep their ribs from breaking.

(Photo by Walt Beazley. Used with permission of University of Tulsa Athletics.)

Not Just for Athletes

Professional athletes were the first to embrace core conditioning as a part of their regular workout routines. As with most things, once the pros do it, everybody jumps on the bandwagon. In this case, that's awesome. Everybody should be training their core because everybody uses their core. You may not realize it, but your core is working right now—even if you're sitting down. The core muscles help with movement and stabilization, but they also help with posture. One of the biggest health complaints today is low-back pain. The number one reason for low-back pain is poor core muscle strength. The deep core muscles of the trunk have been ignored for far too long, and many people are paying the price (and pain can be expensive).

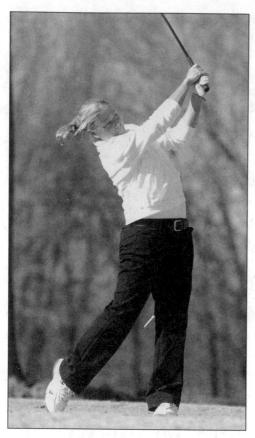

A big difference between a professional and an amateur golfer is the power of their core.

(Photo by Walt Beazley. Used with permission of University of Tulsa Athletics.)

Six-Pack Says

If more people trained their core muscles on a regular basis, I would have far fewer patients complaining of chronic back pain. Most of their pain is caused by weakness.

—Dave Wagon, chiropractor

If athletes can improve their sports performance through core conditioning, imagine what it can do for you. You may not play any sports, but life is often just as challenging. Many of the movements we do every day require a lot of coordination and work from our core. Every time you get the groceries out of the trunk of your car, every time you reach up to get a box off the top shelf, every time you turn around to see who just called out your name, you use your core muscles. It just makes sense to train the muscles you need every day. If your daily activities were just a little bit easier, wouldn't it be worth it? You bet it would. Core conditioning is the answer—and it's a lot more fun than heavy bench presses.

The Least You Need to Know

◆ Your core includes all the muscles of your trunk, including your abs and lower back.

◆ Core conditioning is part of a well-rounded exercise program that includes weight training, body sculpting, aerobic training, and flexibility.

◆ Functional training is another term often used for core conditioning.

◆ You won't necessarily see the results of core training in the mirror because most of the muscles you use are deep inside the body and are covered by other bigger muscles.

◆ Yoga and Pilates are different from core conditioning. They incorporate more flexibility and less power, speed, and aerobic training.

◆ Everyone should include core conditioning as part of their workouts. It's not just for athletes anymore.

In This Chapter

- ◆ Act or react? Muscles that move
- ◆ Your body's core muscles: abdominals, back, and hips
- ◆ Strong bones for a strong body
- ◆ 3D exercise

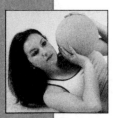 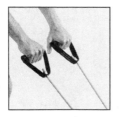 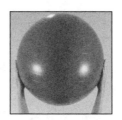 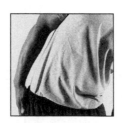 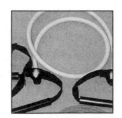 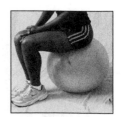

Chapter 2

Core Anatomy

Have you ever stopped to think about how your body works? With more than 100 muscles and 200 bones, there's a lot going on every time you get up and move. Physicians and scientists have spent years studying how the body works, and we still don't know everything. What we do know is that there are certain muscles that make certain movements happen, and certain bones that tie all those muscles together. In the context of core conditioning, we can narrow it down to just a handful of muscles and bones and movements—all of them very important. In fact, if we removed just one of these core muscles from your body, you would basically come to a standstill; movement would become virtually impossible (or at least very, very, very hard).

This chapter introduces you to the anatomy of your core. Don't worry; this won't be as boring as your high school biology class. I'm going to show you how your body works, what muscles and bones are involved, and how it's all integrated to make you one incredible machine. When you're done here, you can impress your friends with your intricate anatomical knowledge—plus understand what these exercises are all about.

Act or React

The debate that probably started the core conditioning craze was whether the muscles of your core acted to make you move, or reacted because you moved. Confused? Most people still are. It's been impossible to define exactly what causes some of the core muscles to activate—but we know that they do. While you are doing the exercises in this book, you will be making certain muscles work because you "told them to." This is called *voluntary movement*. The muscles work because your brain sent a message to them saying, "Hey guys, Bill here wants to get up, so get moving and help him off the couch" (that's the technical jargon).

Involuntary movements are the result of other movements. For instance, when you take a step forward, your torso rotates just slightly to help you stay in balance. You don't have to think about rotating your hips back and forth while you walk; you almost don't have to think about walking. An involuntary movement happens because the body realizes that it needs some help either moving or stabilizing parts of your body. It decides to activate these muscles to keep everything working correctly. Most of the time, you won't even notice or feel these muscles. It's all very top-secret, covert stuff.

Getting Defined

Voluntary movements are actions that you decide to make, such as when you turn the page in this book. Your brain sends the message to the muscles in your arm and hand to turn the page. **Involuntary movements** happen all by themselves when the body and brain decide that they need to happen. You don't have any control over involuntary actions.

In training the core, some muscles will be activated, and some will react to that activation. You really don't need to think about which individual muscles to activate; your higher brain functions will take care of that for you (that's why your brain is there). All you have to do is get your body moving in the right direction to start and then practice the motions described in each exercise; the learning comes automatically. Your body will get itself into motion if you just give it the push it needs to get started. So how about the debate over action or reaction? Who cares, just as long as it all works right!

Muscles of the Core

If you look in the mirror, you might be able to see about 10 to 12 different muscles on the surface of your core. If you were able to strip away muscle layers, you would find that there are actually more than 30 different muscles that are part of or are connected to your core. Can you imagine trying to coordinate 30 different muscles all at one time? Talk about multitasking. That's why we have involuntary muscles; we are incapable of voluntarily controlling that many muscles all at one time.

Six-Pack Says

The most fascinating thing about the body is that it is able to control itself. If our brains had to think about every little muscle that was working during a movement, we'd have a meltdown.
—Lisa Korpela, anatomical biologist

The easiest way to describe muscle anatomy is to break it down into areas of the body and the movements they perform. This is where the scientist in me comes out. I have to tell you about the anatomy, but I'm going to try to do it without putting you to sleep (because sleep is not a core-conditioning exercise).

Abdominals

Your abdominals are actually four separate muscles. The only one that most people look for is the "six-pack" muscle known as the rectus abdominis. Although this is a great-looking muscle, it cannot work alone. It does only one thing: helps you bend forward when you do a crunch. The other three abdominal muscles are equally important because the whole group of them works as a team when you move. The internal and external obliques help you rotate the trunk, and the transversus abdominis is the muscle that works the most when you suck in your stomach.

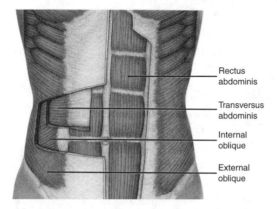

Rectus abdominis

Transversus abdominis

Internal oblique

External oblique

The abdominal muscles are responsible for helping you rotate, bend forward, and suck in your stomach.

The abdominal muscles can also be used to help stabilize your spine. Because the only bones between the bottom of your ribs and the top of your hips are the small vertebrae in back, the abdominal muscles pull double duty in acting kind of like bones. They help define your stomach and "abdominal cavity," where a lot of your internal organs are located. The strength of the abdominals protects these organs and helps stabilize the spine when you are moving and exercising.

Back

There are more muscles in the back and along the spine than anywhere else in the core. The reason is because of all the bones of the spine (the vertebrae) that have to be controlled. The back muscles are often divided into upper-, middle-, and lower-back, depending on what exercise is being used. In real life, or in a real body, the muscles are so interconnected that dividing them into groups is really not possible.

Your lower back is the most susceptible to injury because it relies on muscles and the five lumbar vertebrae to provide most of its protection. These muscles and bones aren't very strong by themselves, which is why core conditioning is more of a holistic approach than a one-muscle-at-a-time type of training. The major muscles of the lower back actually start at the hips and run all the way up to the back of your skull. These are probably the longest muscles in your body, and they overlap each other like the strands in a rope so that their strength is enhanced.

Don't Throw It Out

It's interesting that the most common muscle complaint is a lower-back problem. There are more muscles in the lower back than any other area of the body. The key to a healthy back is a strong back.

Collectively known as the erector spinae, the iliocostalis, longissimus, and spinalis muscles are mainly responsible for keeping your back straight (hence the "erect" part of the name). These muscles are assisted by muscles even deeper in the back, close to the spine. The muscles of your lower back and vertebrae are part of your core musculature, and most of them are involuntary. These muscles are working all the time (except when you are asleep), fighting against gravity. When gravity starts winning, you start hunching over. Ever wonder why some older people are so bent-over? It's in part the fault of weak erector spinae and deep posterior muscles in the back. I'm not going to go into each of the muscles individually because they don't work individually. The exercises you learn later will describe which of these muscle groups is being worked. For now, just check out the pictures here—and don't worry, there won't be a spelling test later.

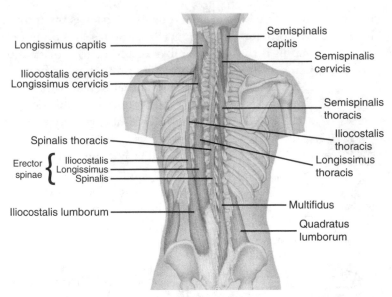

Longissimus capitis

Iliocostalis cervicis
Longissimus cervicis

Spinalis thoracis

Erector
spinae { Iliocostalis
Longissimus
Spinalis

Iliocostalis lumborum

Semispinalis capitis

Semispinalis cervicis

Semispinalis thoracis

Iliocostalis thoracis

Longissimus thoracis

Multifidus

Quadratus lumborum

The muscles in your lower back are mainly responsible for keeping you upright and protecting the spine.

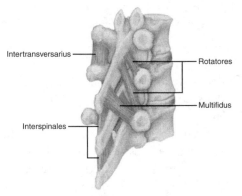

Intertransversarius

Interspinales

Rotatores

Multifidus

These muscles help keep your vertebrae in line and assist in stabilization during most exercises.

Hips

Picture your hips as a transition point between your trunk and your legs. The hips aren't part of your back, aren't part of your abdominals, and really aren't part of your legs. They are a section of anatomy all by themselves, with their own muscles and chores and a life all their own. If you ask someone to name a muscle in their hips, the most common answer is the gluteus maximus. That's actually a good answer because the glutes (including the maximus and the lesser-known gluteus medius and minimus) are the largest muscles in the hips and, therefore, have a lot of responsibility.

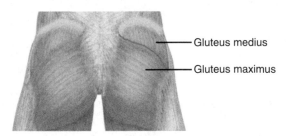

Gluteus medius

Gluteus maximus

The strong glute muscles make up the hip extensors.

The hips move in four ways. You can bend forward, backward, left, and right. Each of these movements originates in the hips, and each movement is caused in part by some muscle in the hip. The glutes are mainly responsible for helping you stand up straight and extend your legs away from your body, also known as hip extension.

On the other side, the rectus femoris, tensor fasciae latae (not a coffee drink), pectineus, iliopsoas, and sartorius muscles help you to bend forward or lift your knee in the air, also known as hip flexion. Finally, there are seven minor muscles that generate a lot of hip rotation (all of which have really long names, so just look at the picture). You'll need these because a lot of the exercises later require a good deal of rotation and power.

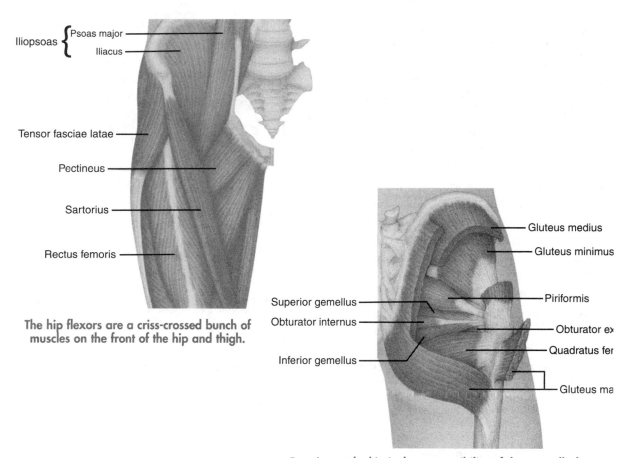

The hip flexors are a criss-crossed bunch of muscles on the front of the hip and thigh.

Rotation at the hip is the responsibility of these small, deep muscles with really long names.

Except for the gluteus maximus and a small part of the gluteus medius, most of the hip muscles are deep inside your body, hidden under other leg muscles so you can't feel them. You'll have to trust me when I say they are in there. If you were missing any of these muscles, you'd probably be walking like a mummy.

More Than a Stack of Bones

Holding up all these muscles is an arrangement of 24 bones collectively called your vertebrae. They are divided into cervical (7 bones), thoracic (12 bones), and lumbar (5 bones) sections. Below these are your sacrum and coccyx, which are portions of fused vertebrae that we aren't really concerned with because they don't play a large part in the movement of the spine.

Your spine is a work of art (mostly abstract). It seems like a really complex design, and it is. Each vertebra is separated from the vertebrae above and below it by a cushioned disc that enables the vertebrae to move in all directions. You can bend, twist, and flex your vertebrae in an infinite number of ways; it truly is a three-dimensional structure.

As you can see from this picture, your spine is not a perfectly straight stack of bones. In fact, it has three distinct curves built into it. When we sit up straight, our spine is actually curved. It's supposed to be that way, and to straighten it any further would really put a kink in your back (did you get the oxymoron there?). All those muscles we discussed earlier are connected to this stack of funny-looking bones at those little stubs you see sticking off the sides of each one. When those muscles contract and pull, the vertebrae they are connected to move in that direction. For instance, if the muscles on the right side of your back pull down, your vertebrae

flexes to the right and you lean over sideways. It's a great contraption that works very well if you keep those muscles strong and flexible.

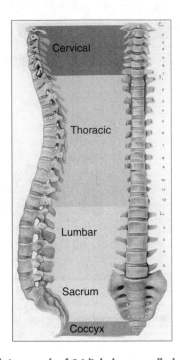

Your back is a stack of 24 little bones called vertebrae.

Moving in Three Directions at Once

Our bodies are three-dimensional objects. We have height, width, and depth. You may not be happy with your height, width, or depth, but you have them anyway. The directions you can move come in three dimensions as well. You can bend forward and backward, you can move side to side, and you can rotate. In technical terms, these are called your frontal, sagittal, and transverse planes. Why is this important? Because if you can exercise in more than one direction at a time, you will see results from your exercise program a whole lot faster. The advanced exercises later in this book involve a lot of three-dimensional exercises in which you move through a little bit of each dimension with each exercise. The more dimensions you can throw into an exercise, the more challenging it becomes and the faster your body responds.

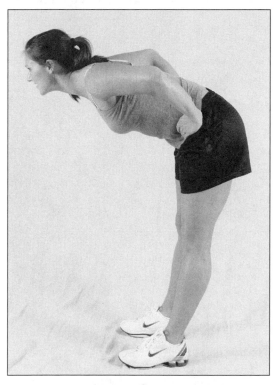

Bending forward (also called forward flexion) is in the frontal plane.

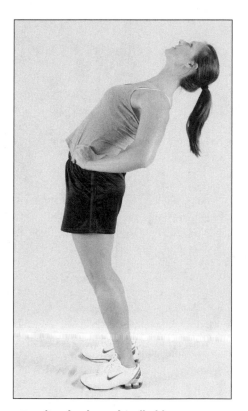

Bending backward (called hyperextension) is also in the frontal plane.

Core conditioning is perfect for three-dimensional exercises because your spine moves in all three directions. Your arms and legs don't like to rotate very much, so most of that movement is left to the spine. With other types of exercise, such as body sculpting or weight lifting, you pretty much stay away from rotation. Without rotation, you are working in only two dimensions, or getting only two thirds of a full workout. That's why core conditioning is so different and so beneficial: your body works in every way it was designed to.

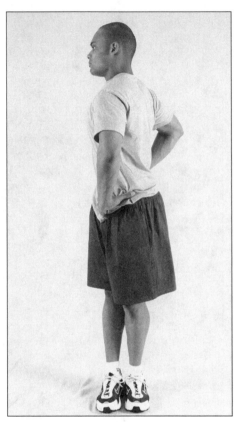

Twisting to the left or right is called rotation in the transverse plane.

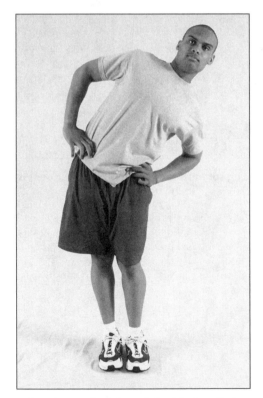

Leaning to the left or right side is called lateral flexion in the sagittal plane.

The Least You Need to Know

- Some muscles are under your voluntary control, and others work when the body tells them to.

- Core conditioning helps train those muscles that you can't see or voluntarily contract.

- Core conditioning is designed to work more than 30 muscles in your trunk.

- The muscles of your back are all integrated and work together to keep your spine in line.

- Your spine is a stack of 24 vertebrae, all tied together with a complex arrangement of muscles.

- Moving in more than one direction at a time helps your body condition itself faster than other types of workouts.

In This Chapter

- ◆ Before you get started …
- ◆ Fitting core conditioning into your workout
- ◆ Training by the numbers
- ◆ New toys for building a new body

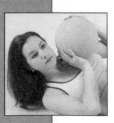
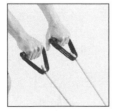
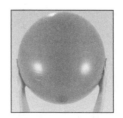
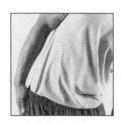
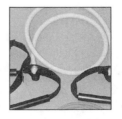
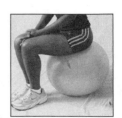

Start with the Basics

Since you've made it this far in the book, I'm guessing that you agree core conditioning is an excellent idea. I stated earlier that core conditioning is something that everyone should do, but the question that still remains is, how do you fit core conditioning into your lifestyle?

Everyone has different demands on their time. You may have a 9-to-5 job that actually takes 8-to-6. You may have kids to shuttle around, schedules to coordinate, and meals to cook. One of the advantages of core conditioning is that it can be done just about anytime and anywhere. For those of you already involved in an exercise program, this chapter shows you how to incorporate the core training exercises of this book into your current workout. If you have never done any core conditioning, it's not a problem; most people haven't, so we talk a little about what you should do first, second, and third. You'll leave this chapter confident that you can work this style of training into your life and become stronger and fitter than you have ever experienced.

Get a Tune-Up

You would never jump in your car and head out for a road trip without making sure the car had plenty of oil, gas, and good tread on the tires. You should treat your body the same way. Before you start asking it to do special core-conditioning exercises—or any new type of exercise training—make sure everything "under the hood" is working well. Make an appointment with your doctor to get a physical if you haven't had one in the last year. Because core conditioning targets the muscles of the back and involves moving the spine a lot, if you have any back problems, ask your doctor or chiropractor if these exercises will be safe for you.

> **Don't Throw It Out**
>
> In the past, I've had to send clients home for the day because their blood pressure was too high. When you exercise, your blood pressure normally rises. If you start out with high blood pressure, it will get even higher—sometimes dangerously high. High blood pressure can't be seen or felt, in most cases. You may look and feel completely fine, but your body may not be working optimally inside. Always have your blood pressure checked before beginning a core-conditioning program.

Additionally, if you have had heart problems, metabolic diseases, or pulmonary issues (including asthma) in the past, get your doctor's clearance before beginning core conditioning. During core-conditioning exercises a lot of stress is placed on the heart. This isn't aerobic training, but your heart rate can get pretty high during some of the advanced exercises—and even during some of the beginning exercises, if this is all new to you.

If you check out okay and everything is running well, there is no reason you can't incorporate core conditioning into your daily life. You are gassed up and ready to hit the road.

Starting from Scratch

The exercises you'll read about later are divided into chapters, based on their difficulty. The beginning exercises are, of course, easier to perform than the advanced exercises. If you are not exercising regularly right now and core conditioning will be your first step toward a better body, start by learning all the beginning exercises before moving on to the more difficult ones. If you are one of those people who thinks that conquering the hardest exercise means you don't need the easier ones, you are in for a big surprise.

The beginning exercises were picked because they teach your body how to use the smaller core muscles instead of the larger surface muscles. If the advanced exercises are done first, without learning how to use your body correctly, the big surface muscles will be contracted and will end up doing more work than you want them to, giving you fewer core-conditioning results than you expected.

Core conditioning is a step-by-step learning process. You have to teach yourself how to move correctly and how to use the proper muscles to create those movements. The best way to accomplish this is by working your way through the beginning exercises until you really feel comfortable with how they work and how they make your body feel. Only then should you move on to the advanced exercises. It's a lot like the old saying "You have to learn to crawl before you learn to walk."

On the same note, you should start with only a few exercises—say, one from each chapter—and build your workout routine slowly. When you start to engage muscles that you haven't focused on before, the usual result is a little bit of initial soreness. I'm telling you this now so you won't be cussing me out later. Any time you start a new exercise routine, a little bit of soreness is to be expected. After all, you are asking muscles that have just been sitting around to get up and get moving. Believe me, they are going to fight back.

If you do just a few exercises initially, the soreness will be minimal and you will quickly get over it. Then you can add more exercises. However, if you jump in with both feet instead of just dipping a toe in first, you'll probably be really sore and have a hard time moving the next day. New exercise routines should be built slowly and carefully. Allowing your body to get used to one new thing before heaping on more will keep you focused on the positive outcome of the program and help prevent potential injuries.

Six-Pack Says

Doing too much too fast usually leads to doing nothing at all.

—Jay Dawes, One-Eighty Personal Training

As you pick exercises to start your new program, don't just pick the ones that look neat. Start at the beginning of the chapter and try out each exercise. Find the ones that you really like, that you really feel, and that really make you work. The best exercises are usually the ones that we don't want to do because they're difficult. Conquering these harder exercises means that your body is responding and adapting, getting stronger and more conditioned. It's okay to play with the easy exercises, but don't rely on them to transform your body. It's never quite that simple. Think of it like this: if it's easy, your body doesn't have to work hard enough to make any changes, so you'll basically be wasting your time. A little later in the chapter, I cover exactly how much to do and when to do it.

Adding Core Conditioning to Your Workout

For all you seasoned exercise buffs out there, adding core conditioning to an already full workout session may seem difficult. How can you fit more exercises into your already taxing workouts? Well, you can stay at the gym longer and avoid going home, or you can make core conditioning a functional part of your workout and actually get more done in less time.

Here's a little science experiment for you. Visit your favorite gym and count the number of people actually working and the number of people sitting around. Based on my own observations, at any one time, probably 75 percent of the people I watch in the gym are sitting around "resting" between sets. I agree that rest is important, but it's rare that your entire body needs to rest at the same time—we usually call that *sleep*. Core conditioning can be integrated into your workout during those rest periods between your other exercises. Instead of sitting and catching your breath between sets of bicep curls, get down on the floor and do a core-conditioning exercise. As long as you aren't using those bicep muscles, they are still getting the rest they need while you are getting more done in the same amount of time.

The key to this method is to pick core-conditioning exercises that don't involve the same muscles that you are using during your body-sculpting or weight-lifting exercises. When you are doing sets for your legs, use core-conditioning exercises that focus on your core and upper body. When you work your upper body, choose core-conditioning exercises that target your hips, abs, and lower back. Rest doesn't have to mean sitting down and doing nothing; it just means that a certain part of your body is resting.

By the Numbers

By now, I'm sure you are wondering exactly how much core conditioning you are going to have to do to see any difference. The first thing to remember is that you may not "see" any difference, but you will most likely "feel" the difference. So how much does it take to feel the difference? Not much. Truth be told, you will feel improvements from doing just one of these exercises every day—but that will take you only so far.

You can take a couple of different approaches to your core-conditioning workout. You can dedicate an entire session to core conditioning, or you can integrate core conditioning into another exercise program, such as body sculpting. Whichever way you choose, here are some general rules to follow.

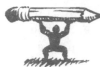

Suck It In _____

If you're interested in learning more about body sculpting, see my book *The Complete Idiot's Guide to Body Sculpting Illustrated* (Alpha Books, 2004).

More Than Three Minutes a Day

I wish getting in shape were as simple as those television infomercials make it look. If we could get by with just three minutes of exercise every day, the whole world would be walking around with rock-hard muscles, lean bodies, and super-model looks. It seems like every time you turn on the TV, there is another "super-secret, state-of-the-art, just-discovered miracle exercise" that promises to turn a flabby body into solid muscle in just a few minutes each day. What they don't tell you is that those three minutes of a single exercise are usually just part of an overall exercise program that should also include core conditioning, weight lifting, cardiovascular exercise, flexibility training, and proper nutrition (they put all of that in the fine print, right next to "Results shown are not typical").

If any of what they say on those infomercials were true, gyms would be out of business, everyone would look great, and this book would be only five pages long. Unfortunately, that miracle exercise is yet to be discovered—and probably never will be. Your body is far too complicated for any one exercise to involve all the different muscles, bones, and joints in your body. It simply can't be done.

Now I'm not saying that you have to spend hours every day on your core-conditioning program, but it's definitely going to take more than 3 minutes. In reality, you can get your entire core training finished in 20 to 30 minutes. What's even better is that you don't have to do it all at once. That's really the best part of core conditioning. If you don't have 30 minutes to dedicate

to this exercise program, set aside three 10-minute sessions each day, or six 5-minute sessions each day. Do a few exercises in the morning and a couple at lunch, and finish after dinner. Doing a few minutes of core-conditioning exercise spread throughout your day has the same effect as doing all your exercises at one time.

Your body doesn't care if every muscle is working at the same time. Improvements come from the accumulation of all the exercise you do, not just one particular session at a certain time of the day. There is no magic effect of wearing yourself out all at once. All that does is make it harder for you to move on to the next task in your busy schedule.

Find a time, or times, that works best for you. The key is really just getting it done, regardless of when you do it. As I mentioned earlier, for you seasoned workout buffs, fitting core conditioning into your existing program can be as simple as doing one exercise in between each of your current exercises. You can dedicate a full session just to core conditioning, or you can do it as part of each daily workout. You may even have days when you don't do any core conditioning (yes, it's okay to take a day off now and then).

The best-case scenario for all of us is to do 30 minutes every day. I know that may not be possible for everyone, so do what you can now and think of 30 minutes as your goal. A minimum of three times a week will get you some fast results. Any less than twice a week won't produce any noticeable changes, so rearrange your schedule and fit in a little core conditioning as often as possible.

Sets, Reps, and Weights

Core-conditioning exercises are different from other types of exercises in more than one way. Sure, they look different and work different muscles, but how much you do of them is a little unusual as well. Core exercises don't always have predetermined numbers of sets and repetitions (reps for short). On top of that, you aren't going to be using barbells or dumbbells, so the weights are added up a little differently.

Each of the exercises in the following chapters includes a description of how many sets and reps to do, and how to adjust the intensity of the exercise. Because core conditioning is more about completing motions than it is about lifting a certain amount of weight, the sets and reps are more guidelines than hard rules. I've provided you with a goal number of sets and reps for each exercise; you then have to work up to that goal. If you can do only one set to begin with, that's fine. Don't push yourself to finish just because I said so. Listen to your body and do only as much as you are able to.

The best rule to follow in core conditioning is that proper form is the best indicator of how much to do. When you start losing proper form, you're done for the session. Because many of the muscles you will be using during these exercises are out of your conscious control (meaning you can't voluntarily contract them just by thinking about them), you have to be conscious of your form instead. When your form falters, your ability to do the exercise decreases and the chance of injury increases.

Don't Throw It Out

Maintaining proper form during each repetition of each exercise is the key to making injury-free improvements. Never sacrifice form just to get in a couple more reps; the risk outweighs the benefit.

Some of these exercises are done for a specified length of time instead of repetitions. A set may be only one repetition of 15–20 seconds, or one repetition of up to 60 seconds. During these exercises, a goal time is given for you to work up to. This goal time (say, 60 seconds) is the longest amount of time you should perform an exercise without rest. Going beyond this goal time won't provide you with much more benefit. This is based on the principle of diminishing returns. There is a point at which doing more of an exercise actually provides fewer results. I've already calculated these times for you; your job is to work up to the maximum goal time and then maintain that level of fitness. As an example, doing 90 seconds instead of 60 seconds doesn't mean that your results will be 50 percent greater; actually, they will be only 5–10 percent greater, if even that much.

The energy systems your body uses to fuel these exercises also have a limited supply. Once you use up that supply (usually within 60 seconds), you won't be able to continue the exercise correctly and your body won't be able to fuel itself correctly. This is when you rest.

As for weight, core conditioning has the distinction of being one of the easiest forms of exercise to complete because you don't need much equipment. In most cases, your body weight is all that you need to get the core muscles involved and working hard. As you'll see in a moment, there isn't any heavy iron or steel involved. No more adding up the number of iron plates! In core-conditioning exercises, the weight is often measured by the size of a medicine ball, the amount of stretch in the resistance tubing, how your body is positioned during the exercise, and how fast you do the exercise.

Your core muscles are essentially controlling the levers of your body—your arms and legs. You can place your body in particular positions that make the core muscles more active by changing how far away the resistance is from your core. For instance, if you hold this book against your chest, it seems really light. However, if you hold it out in front of you away from your body, it feels much heavier. The weight of the book hasn't changed, but it feels heavier because it is farther away from your core and those core muscles are working harder. You use this principle of physics to change the intensity of each exercise without having to add bulky weights to your workout (I'll bet you didn't know you were going to learn about physics in this book).

How fast you do an exercise can change the intensity as well. Sometimes you will be instructed to do an exercise very slowly, to give the muscles time to work. Other times you will be told to move as fast as you can. This makes the muscles contract faster and produce more force. Each speed (faster or slower) has its own advantages, depending on the exercise. Some exercises, such as abdominal crunches (see Chapter 4), should never be done fast. Likewise, exercises such as the forward chop (see Chapter 6) have to be done fast, or you won't get the full benefit. Faster isn't always harder; it depends on the type of exercise you are doing and the particular muscles you are targeting. Follow the guidelines for each exercise to make sure you are performing it at the correct speed.

Overall, core conditioning is one of the simplest exercise prescriptions for me to give. All you have to do is follow the recommendations on the correct number of sets, repetitions, and weight for each exercise, and I guarantee that you will find yourself making great progress while staying injury-free.

Six-Pack Says

Just as you can't judge a book by its cover, you can't judge the effectiveness of an exercise by how much weight is being used. Core conditioning may look simple on the outside, but your muscles are working like crazy on the inside.

—Becki Lea, fitness model

Progression and Planning

The following chapters detail more than a hundred different core-conditioning exercises. Deciding which exercises are right for you is a little more complicated than just flipping through the pages and randomly stopping somewhere because a picture looks cool. Because most of the pictures in this book show really cool exercises, I'm going to make it super easy for you to choose the best exercises for your body.

As I've said before, start with the beginning exercises, and get really good and comfortable with them before moving on to the advanced exercises. So which beginning exercises should you use? Easy—start at the front of a chapter and work your way through it, exercise by exercise. Not only is this book divided into beginning and advanced exercises, but each exercise in each chapter is organized according to difficulty. For example, in Chapter 4, begin with the abdominal crunch before moving on to the oblique crunch; then try out the reverse crunch. Just follow the order of exercises in each chapter, and everything should go smoothly.

Besides choosing the right exercises, an important part of any exercise program is doing just the right amount. Your body will improve only when it has to do more work than it is normally used to doing. This is the principle of progression. Your body will adapt if you force it to adapt. Otherwise, bodies are very lazy and will just stay the same. If you make yours work, it will change. Proper progression is as simple as doing as much as you can with proper form and then trying a little more during the next workout. You should always be able to move forward, completing more each workout (even if it's just a couple more seconds or one more repetition). If you ever can't do as much as you did in your last workout, you haven't rested enough.

The proper amount of rest between workouts is 48 hours, or every other day. You can work out every day; you just can't do the same exercises every day. Your body has to have some time to recuperate and let those muscles you just worked get ready for the next workout. It takes at least 48 hours to do this, sometimes 72 hours (3 days). You have to listen to your body and push it just enough, but not too much. I wish there were an exact number I could give you to follow here, but everybody is a little different, so you have to pay attention to how you feel before you begin another workout. It's all about planning ahead.

Suck It In

If you plan your workouts in advance, knowing which exercises you are going to do on which days, you will have a general game plan to follow. You may not stick to that plan perfectly—few plans are perfect—but if you listen to how your body feels, pushing yourself just a little further each day, you can count on seeing steady improvements in your core fitness level.

As I stated earlier, each exercise has a goal number of sets and repetitions (or time). Start by completing as many sets and repetitions as you feel comfortable with (but don't stop just when it's getting hard). Each exercise should challenge you but not hurt you. If you work to the point that it hurts to do another rep, you've gone too far. I suggest erring on the side of caution by doing too little in the beginning instead of too much. As you learn how much you can handle and get comfortable with an exercise, you will know how hard you can push yourself and be safe.

Keep track of your workouts by using a simple log book. Write down what exercises you completed, how many sets and reps you finished,

and how much rest you took. Also tracking how you felt after each workout can give you clues as to how your body is responding each time you change your routine a little bit. Refer to your log book before each workout so you know exactly where to pick up and what to shoot for. A sample log page is shown in Appendix C.

When you have worked your way up to the goal of each exercise, all you have to do is maintain that level of fitness. Maintaining is a lot easier than improving. To maintain a level of fitness, continue to complete all the sets and reps of that exercise, but do it only once a week. To move beyond maintenance, choose the next-hardest exercise in that chapter, or a variation on that exercise, if it's available, and start working on learning it.

There are enough exercises and variations in this book to keep your workouts changing for several years to come. Check out the sample workout plans in Appendix C for some ideas to get you going and staying on track.

The Tools

As I mentioned in Chapter 1, core conditioning has got to be one of the most portable forms of exercise there is. Sure, there are gyms almost everywhere you go, and jogging is always an option, but to really get a good core-conditioning workout, you never even have to leave the comfort of your air-conditioned home (or hotel room, if you are traveling). One time I even did my entire core-conditioning workout on an airplane during a 5-hour flight. You don't have to have a lot of room, and you need virtually no equipment at all to get everything you need from this type of exercise plan.

To Gym or Not to Gym?

I don't want to discourage you from joining a quality health club or gym. If fact, many exercises do require the special equipment that only commercial gyms can provide. Your body-sculpting or weight-training program will probably require access to barbells, dumbbells, and exercise machines to complete all those special exercises—but not core conditioning. You don't have to join a gym, have a special exercise room at home, or own any expensive equipment to get started. As you progress, you will need some minimal equipment, but nothing big and heavy. All the equipment you need for a great core-conditioning workout can be carried around in a small gym bag or backpack. When I train clients in their homes, I bring everything I need, including the equipment I'm about to show you, in a duffel bag slung over my shoulder.

> **Six-Pack Says** _____
>
> There aren't enough gyms in the world to accommodate everybody who needs to work out, because that's everybody.
> —Jimmy Little, health club owner

Some of the more advanced exercises are best done in a gymnasium or outside, where there's more room to move around, but you still don't have to join a club to do these. In each exercise description, I detail what you need and how much room you need. A few exercises involve throwing a ball, so these are best done outside or in a big, open room. Other than that, all you need is a small, empty space to get your workout going.

Real Equipment

You need only three pieces of equipment to do every exercise in this book: resistance tubing, a medicine ball, and a stability ball. That's it. Not a single piece of heavy iron in the list—and, no, I'm not trying to sell you on some super-secret piece of exercise equipment that will do everything you ever dreamed of. In fact, these three types of equipment have been around for a long time and have been used for many different forms of exercise by many different types of people. They just happen to fit into our goals for core conditioning as well.

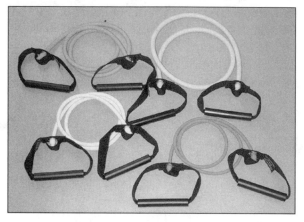

Resistance tubing comes in several different sizes. The thicker it is, the more intense the workout will be.

In the beginning, there were long, Slinky-like springs that could be stretched to provide resistance during exercise. Somebody got the idea that a big rubber band could do the same thing and never rust from the sweat that gets on it. Another person took the rubber band idea and came up with hollow tubing that is far less likely to snap in half when it's stretched. So today we have this high-tech surgical tubing with handles on each end that we call resistance tubing. Aside from the handles, the really neat thing about tubing is that you can vary the resistance by using a different thickness of tubing or by using a shorter or longer tube. The thicker the tubing is, the more intense an exercise becomes. Likewise, if you shorten the length of the tubing, it gets harder. The tubing is infinitely adjustable, unlike any dumbbell ever made. To make it even better, it weighs only a few ounces and can be rolled up and stuffed in your briefcase or purse to carry with you wherever you go.

If that sounded like an infomercial pitch, I apologize. I just can't get over how cool resistance tubing is. If you've never tried it, you've got to get some now. When you are trying to decide which level of tubing to buy, they are often listed as "easy," "light," "medium," "hard," and "very hard," or something similar. There is no way to put a number on how "heavy" tubing is because it all depends on how far you stretch it. My advice is to get two or three different sizes. Some exercises will need more resistance than others, and as you progress, you will need to increase the intensity. You won't ever get to the point that tubing doesn't provide enough resistance. I've had the biggest football players around use resistance tubing and get totally worn-out using it.

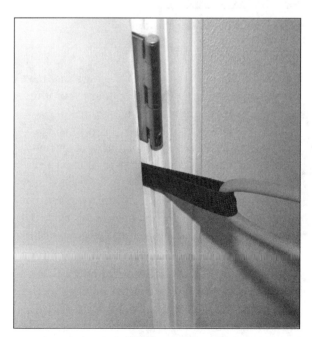

The tubing anchor turns any doorway into the perfect exercise location.

To use resistance tubing anywhere you go, you have to be able to attach one end of it to something solid so you can pull on the other end. If there is a pole, heavy couch, or tree available, you're set. A great piece of equipment to help you set up most of the exercises that use resistance tubing is the tubing door anchor. This is basically a loop of heavy nylon webbing that you stick in the hinge side of any doorway and then close the door, effectively wedging it in place. All you have to do then is thread your tubing through the loop sticking out of the door, and you have a solid anchor.

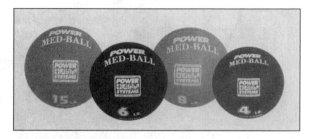

Medicine balls come in different sizes and weights; some bounce and some don't, and some are made of rubber and some of leather.

Medicine balls are probably one of the oldest forms of exercise equipment known to man. If I'm right, in the beginning they were made of rock. They have changed a lot in recent years. Old balls were full of sand and covered in stitched leather. Now they are made of hard rubber and actually bounce like a basketball. You can still get soft ones and balls full of sand, but I don't recommend it. They just don't last as long and are not nearly as versatile. Medicine balls are great for core conditioning because you can hold them in both hands, bounce them, and throw them. They also won't hurt your floor if you drop them, and they provide another form of resistance known as "momentum." When you get a medicine ball moving in one direction, to stop it you have to exert force in the opposite direction. The result is that more muscles work in every exercise you do, which, again, leads to more results from your program.

Medicine balls are sold according to their weight. For you beginners, start with a 5- to 10-pound ball. As you need more resistance, get heavier balls. Probably the heaviest ball you should ever use with any of the exercises in this book is a 20- to 25-pound ball—and that's really heavy.

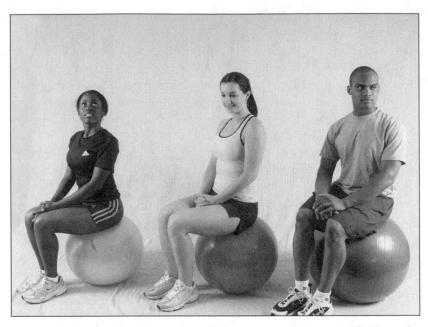

Stability balls typically come in three different sizes. The correct size depends on your height.

Stability balls have been around for only about 20 years, but their popularity has really soared in the last 5 years. Once considered only a tool for physical therapy, stability balls quickly found a place in resistance training because of the vast number of positions and exercises that you can do with them. The correct size of stability ball for you depends on your height. To make sure the ball is the right height for you, when you sit on it, your knees and hips should be at the same height, as shown in the photo. You can also use the following guidelines to determine the right size of ball for you:

- 5 feet and shorter: Use a 45-cm ball
- 5 feet, 1 inch to 5 feet, 6 inches: Use a 55-cm ball
- 5 feet, 7 inches and taller: Use a 65-cm ball

Stability balls don't provide much resistance, but they do provide different forms of leverage.

You will find exercises in later chapters that have you sitting and lying on the ball, and holding the ball with your feet, between your knees, and over your head. The size and give of the ball is what makes it so special: this is an unstable surface that your body has to react to. This is way different from lying on a hard exercise bench. The ball will try to move when you move, so you have to work to prevent that. The resulting effect is that more muscles get involved with each exercise, and you get better results.

See the list of resources in Appendix B for the best places to buy resistance tubing, medicine balls, and stability balls. You can get this stuff at just about any discount sporting goods store, but the quality is often very poor. I always suggest that you spend a little more money in the beginning to get quality equipment that will last two to three times as long as the cheap stuff.

Chapter 3: Start with the Basics   **33**

Your State-of-the-Art Body

The biggest tool you have in your core-conditioning workshop is your own body. A lot of these exercises will make your body work against itself for resistance. If you think about it, each segment of your body has weight. When you move that segment, muscles have to move that weight because that weight is the resistance. If we say your legs weigh 70 pounds, and I ask you to lie down and lift your legs in the air, the core muscles are lifting 70 pounds.

Depending on how you are positioned in any given exercise, your body will always be providing resistance because of your body weight. The one thing you can't control is what happens if you lose weight: that decreases the resistance you have to work with. Although this may be a good argument for gaining weight, I don't recommend it. When you lose weight, you have to compensate by doing more sets or reps in each exercise to keep increasing the resistance. What a wonderful problem to have!

So now that you have a general outline of how much core conditioning you need to do, and you have the tools to do it, it's time to read on to the next chapter and get moving!

The Least You Need to Know

◆ Always get a check-up from your doctor before beginning any new exercise program.

◆ Core-conditioning workouts can be done alone or along with a body-sculpting or weight-training workout.

◆ It takes more than 3 minutes a day to get the results you are after. A good core workout should last about 30 minutes.

◆ Start with the beginning exercises until you can complete the goal number of reps, sets, and time for each one.

◆ You have to push yourself a little further each workout to make your body continually improve.

◆ You don't need a lot of special equipment, or even a gym, to do core conditioning. A gym bag of toys and a small space are all you need to get moving.

In This Part

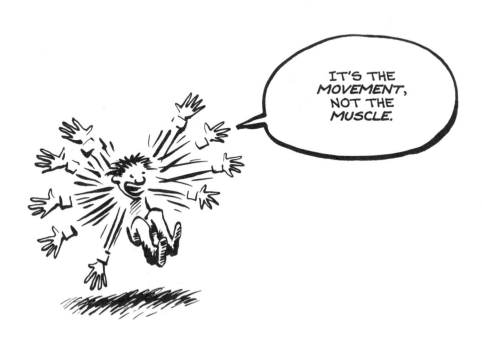

Part 2

Targeting Movements, Not Muscles

Ever thought an exercise looked too complex for you to try? Not anymore. This section of the book is the meat and potatoes (and dessert) of your core-conditioning program. Listed here is every exercise you will ever need to design and keep your core-conditioning program on track. Step-by-step instructions on each exercise, along with accurate pictures of real people doing them, will alleviate any fears you have and leave you feeling energized and excited about what you will be able to do.

In This Chapter

- ◆ Working against gravity
- ◆ Targeting your abdominal and oblique muscles
- ◆ Getting deep back muscles working
- ◆ Adding balance and stabilization

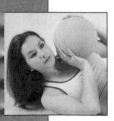
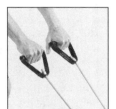
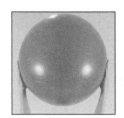
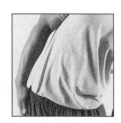
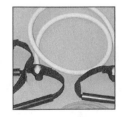
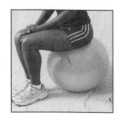

Chapter 4

Beginning Body Weight Resistance

It's all around you, but you can't see it. It pushes on you all the time. It has a speed of 9.8 meters per second squared. The only place to get away from it is in outer space. No, it's not "the force," but kinda: it's gravity! Your body weight is a result of this annoying part of nature that acts upon your body, pushing you down toward the ground all the time. You may as well use it to your advantage.

Your body weight is the result of gravity. Your own body weight is absolutely the most compact and portable form of resistance you can find. You already take it everywhere you go, so there's nothing extra to buy or pack in your suitcase—it's fully functional and really cheap! Gravity has the biggest effect on us when we are standing, and the least effect when we are lying down. Any time you try to leave the floor, gravity tries to push you back down. This provides a source of resistance that you always have to work against, and your core muscles are the main muscles that do that work.

The exercises in this chapter are beginning moves that use only your body weight for the resistance. Some of these exercises you will recognize as tried-and-true movements (which are usually the ones we don't enjoy very much) that can really stimulate the core muscles. Because your body weight doesn't change during an exercise, as you become more fit, you will quickly outgrow these exercises. Once these body weight exercises become too easy, move on to the advanced body weight exercises in the next chapter, and then on to using resistance tubing, medicine balls, and stability balls in the following chapters for a more challenging workout. In a pinch, you can always use these exercises when you are traveling on vacation and want to take it easy but still maintain your core fitness level.

Abdominal Crunch

The abdominal crunch is the granddaddy of all core exercises. The abdominal crunch involves mainly your rectus abdominis (the six-pack part) and your oblique abdominals (right under the "love handles"). Most core-conditioning exercises go after the unseen deep muscles of the trunk, but there are also a few muscles that are on the surface. This exercise helps you get that cut-up six-pack look, but its true advantage is that it strengthens the stomach muscles and helps to provide stability for many of the advanced exercises you will do later in this book. The abdominal crunch is really the first half of the old sit-up, but it doesn't require a partner or a heavy object to anchor your feet. Of all the exercises you will ever do, the abdominal crunch probably involves the least amount of actual movement—but it packs a punch.

Preparation

1. Lie down on your back on a carpeted surface, or use an exercise mat.
2. Bend your knees and keep your feet flat on the floor. Your heels should be placed no more than a foot away from your butt.
3. Cross your arms over your chest. If you want to put your hands on the side of your head, that's okay as well. However, do not lock your hands together under your head or support your head with your hands.

Movement

4. Take a deep breath in, and as you blow it out, roll your head and shoulders off the ground toward your knees. You have to go up only about 30 degrees, or to the point that you start to feel your shoulder blades leave the ground. Your lower back should stay on the floor.

5. Slowly lower yourself back to the ground, take a new breath in, and repeat the process.

Precautions

◆ If your neck muscles get tired and you feel like your head is getting heavy, rest for a moment. The reason you shouldn't lock your hands behind your head or support your head in any way is that the abdominal crunch is also a good way to strengthen the neck muscles. In the beginning, those neck muscles may be weak and get tired before your abdominals do, so let them rest and then begin exercising after a few breaths. And don't worry—you won't develop a big football player–like neck. You'll just make the muscles already there a bit stronger.

◆ Avoid jerking movements in an attempt to get in a couple more reps. The abdominal muscles like to work in smooth motions, and jerking them can cause the back muscles to contract and spasm.

Variations

There will come a time when you can do crunches until you get totally bored. As the abdominal muscles get stronger, you will need to find other ways to stimulate them to work harder.

Add extra weight to your lift by holding a medicine ball against your chest directly under your chin or out over your head. Be careful not to strain your neck muscles with too much weight. An extra 5–15 pounds of resistance is plenty.

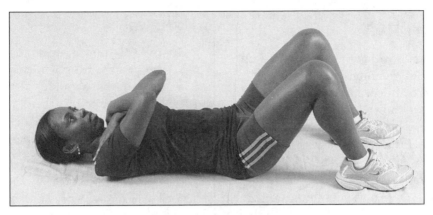

Starting/ending position.

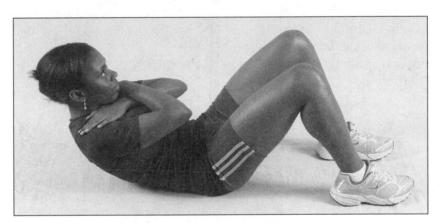

Midpoint position.

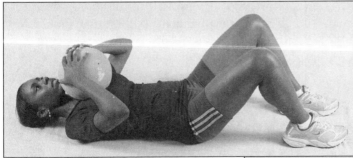

Variation with medicine ball on your chest.

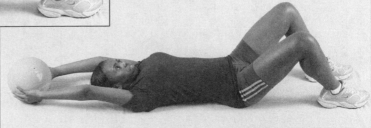

Variation with medicine ball over your head.

Oblique Crunch

The oblique crunch will get you all twisted up. The muscles called the internal and external obliques are the main core muscles that work when you turn around to look behind you. Any time you rotate the body or twist the trunk, these deeper core muscles work along with some of the back muscles that stabilize the vertebrae. Although you really don't feel the oblique muscles contracting as much as you do the larger abdominal muscles, believe me when I say that they are working hard. This exercise will help prepare you for more advanced exercises later that involve rotating your trunk. For now, really concentrate on relaxing the back muscles and letting the internal and external oblique muscles get their groove on.

Preparation

1. Lie down on your back on a carpeted surface, or use an exercise mat.

2. Bend your knees and keep your feet flat on the floor. Your heels should be placed no more than a foot away from your butt.

3. Cross your arms over your chest so your fingers touch your shoulders.

Movement

4. Twist as you roll up so that one shoulder stays on the floor while the other side rolls up until that shoulder blade is off the floor. Remember to breathe out as you lift. It's almost like you are trying to roll over, but your hips and one shoulder are glued to the floor.

5. Lower yourself back to the floor.

6. This exercise works only one side of your body at a time, so you can alternate from side to side; or, you can do a complete set on one side and then go the other way.

Precautions

If you suffer from low-back pain, or if your doctor has told you that you shouldn't twist your body, skip this exercise. When you do oblique crunches, you are also moving your lower vertebrae (the lumbar section) in a twisting fashion. If you experience any pain during this exercise, stop and consult your doctor.

Variations

When you can do oblique crunches without much effort, add some weight to the shoulder being lifted. Hold a medicine ball on that shoulder as you crunch. Five to fifteen pounds is plenty.

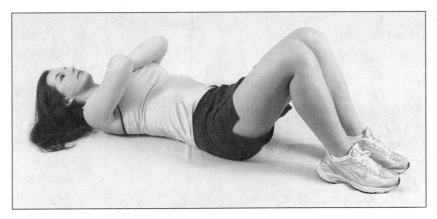

Starting/ending position.

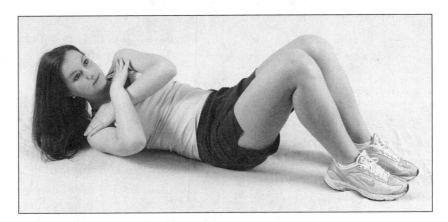

Midpoint position.

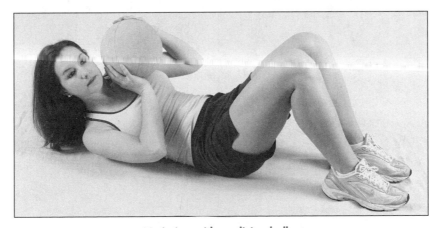

Variation with medicine ball.

Reverse Crunch

The lower part of your abdominal muscles is not stressed very much during abdominal crunches or oblique crunches because the upper part is straining against the weight of your upper body while the lower part is anchoring the exercise. To stress the lower portions of these muscles a little bit harder, we need to do crunches in reverse—a.k.a. butt raises. These are the muscles directly under that belly pooch that many of us complain of, and they are the muscles you will see when you get rid of that extra layer of fat. When you do these correctly, you should feel the "burn" in your lower abs right between your hip bones.

Preparation

1. Lie down on your back on a carpeted surface, or use an exercise mat.

2. Put your hands behind your head and rest your elbows on the floor. Because you aren't going to be raising your head, having your hands behind your head is okay this time.

3. Bend your knees and lift your legs up so it looks like you're sitting in a chair that fell over.

Movement

4. Slowly roll your hips up and off the floor while you breathe out. When done correctly, you'll feel like you're rolling into the fetal position. I like to think about bringing my knees toward my chin, to keep me focused on the movement.

5. Stop rolling up when you feel your lower back start to lift up. You don't want to go any farther than this. Roll up slowly so that momentum doesn't carry you too far. Though the movement is small, it's very beneficial.

6. Slowly lower your hips back to the floor, but keep your legs in the air and ready for the next repetition.

Precautions

It is extremely important that you do this exercise slowly. Do not use momentum to roll yourself up or in an attempt to do a few extra reps. When you use your abdominal muscles, the back muscles should be resting. Jerking or moving too quickly can cause the back muscles to contract, which can end up causing injury.

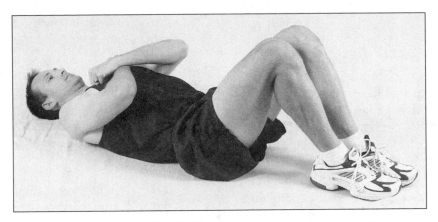

Starting/ending position.

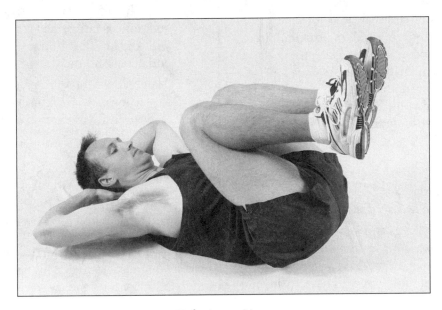

Midpoint position.

Sit-Up

The sit-up is an age-old exercise that has come under a lot of scrutiny in the last 10 years. Many "fitness experts" have advised against the sit-up because it doesn't target the abdominal muscles as well as a straight abdominal crunch does and because it supposedly can hurt your back. There is no proof that the sit-up can cause injury to your back if your back is healthy. In fact, the back muscles aren't even working during a properly performed sit-up. The benefit of a sit-up over an abdominal crunch is that the sit-up also involves the core hip flexor muscles. These are the muscles that help you to lift your leg forward during walking or climbing stairs. After years of not doing sit-ups, most people find them challenging. As your hip-flexor muscles strengthen, this exercise won't be that hard and you will be in better shape than your crunch-only friends.

Preparation

1. Lie down on your back on a carpeted surface, or use an exercise mat.

2. Bend your knees and keep your feet flat on the floor. Your heels should be placed no more than a foot away from your butt. In the beginning, you will have to anchor your feet under a heavy object, such as a couch, or have someone hold your feet down. When you get stronger, you can do this without anchoring your feet.

3. Cross your arms over your chest. If you want to put your hands on the side of your head, that's okay as well. However, do not lock your hands together under your head or support your head with your hands.

Movement

4. Take a deep breath in, and as you blow it out, roll your head and shoulders off the ground toward your knees (this is basically an abdominal crunch so far). When your shoulders leave the floor, keep your abdominals contracted and begin pulling with the hip flexor muscles to bring your entire back all the way off the floor.

5. Touch your elbows to your knees and slowly lower yourself back to the floor. Repeat until your set is complete.

Precautions

When you start to get tired, concentrate on performing the abdominal crunch portion of the sit-up under control. Do not let yourself get into the habit of jerking up off the floor when your abs get tired. This will cause the back muscles to contract and could cause injury.

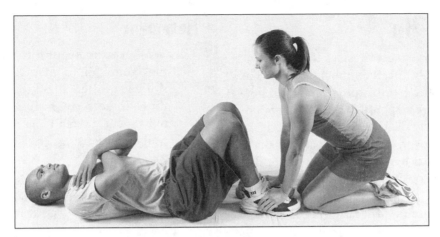

Starting/ending position.

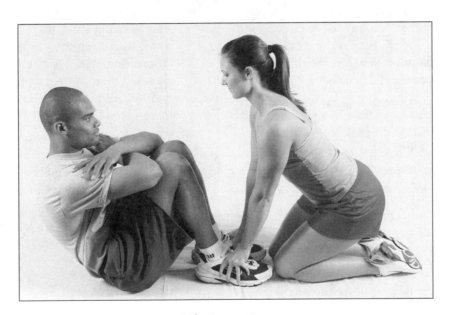

Midpoint position.

Wall Roll-Up

This exercise targets the muscles that perform exactly opposite of the abdominal muscles. The back extensors (or erector spinae and deep posterior muscles) are responsible for keeping your back straight and tall. When you see elderly people stooped over, part of the reason is that the back extensors have lost their strength. Because these are considered "postural" muscles that work all the time, most people overlook them in their training programs (but not you). A solid core-conditioning program will incorporate this exercise and others like it to balance out the strength of the abdominal muscles. In fact, it's essential that you include exercises for your lower back any time you do exercises for your abdominals, to prevent a muscular imbalance from front to back. It's difficult to feel these muscles working, simply because there are not a lot of nerve receptors to provide feedback to your brain. With practice, you will get a good sense of being able to control your movements and these deep muscles.

Preparation

1. Stand with your head, shoulders, and hips against a wall, and your feet about a foot in front of you.

2. Your arms will hang down at your sides for this entire exercise.

Movement

3. While keeping your hips against the wall, tuck your chin to your chest and slowly roll your vertebrae off the wall one at a time. To keep you focused on the correct movement, pretend you are stuck to the wall and are being "peeled off" from the top down.

4. When your entire back is off the wall and only your hips remain in contact with the wall, slowly raise yourself back to the starting position by rolling your back against the wall one vertebrae at a time, starting at your hips and working up. Think of this as being stuck back to the wall. You want to concentrate on moving slowly and "unrolling" your body until it is straight again. The movement of one vertebrae at a time will highlight the activity of the back extensor muscles.

5. When you get your entire back against the wall, raise your head until it rests against the wall, and try to stretch yourself up toward the ceiling, making yourself as tall as possible.

6. Relax your back and begin another repetition.

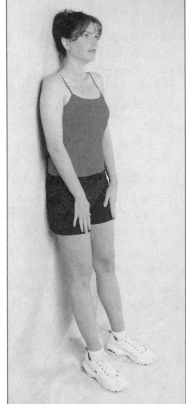

Starting/ending position.

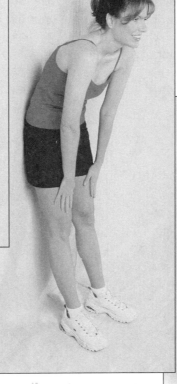

Halfway down position.

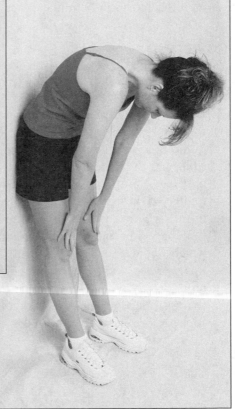

Midpoint position.

Pointer

The pointer exercise adds a touch of balance and coordination to your workout. While doing this exercise, gravity will be trying to force your back into extension (making you look like an old horse with a sagging back). You have to contract one set of muscles to counteract gravity, while using another set of muscles to balance. This adds a level of difficulty, but it is easily mastered with practice. Pay special attention to keeping your back flat, and progress to each level of balance only after you feel comfortable and stable with the first. When you get the hang of this exercise, the more advanced balance exercises later will be much easier.

Preparation

1. Kneel on your hands and knees on either an exercise mat or a carpeted surface.

2. Before starting the movement, you have to get your back into a neutral position. To do this, arch your back as high as possible, and then allow it to sag as low as possible. Neutral position is exactly in the middle of these two extremes. If you are unsure whether you are in a neutral position, have a friend give you directions on which way to move (up or down), or do this exercise next to a mirror so you can monitor yourself. When you are in a neutral position, stay there and don't let your back sag or arch.

Movement

3. The first balance position is done by lifting one arm directly out in front of you. Now you are balancing on one hand and both knees. Practice this position until you feel stable and are not wobbling around.

4. Holding the first balance position (one arm out in front of you), straighten the opposite leg behind you to the second balance position. If your left arm is out, straighten your right leg, and vice versa. Hold this position for up to 60 seconds.

5. Rest for 10–15 seconds, and repeat the balance positions with the other arm and leg so that both sides have a chance to work. Your goal should be five repetitions of 60 seconds on each side. Work your way up to that, and then you'll know you have conquered this exercise.

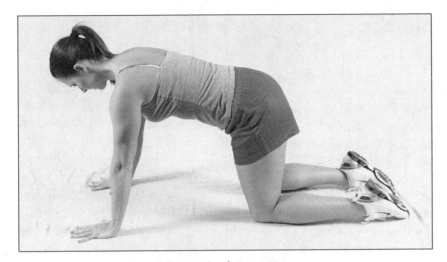

Starting/ending position.

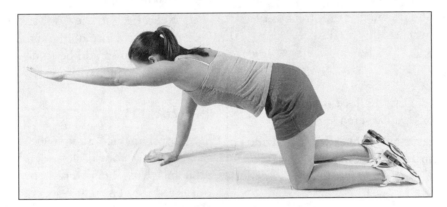

First balance position.

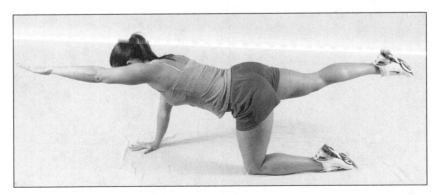

Second balance position.

Flying Superman

The flying Superman is actually done on the ground, so I'm sorry if I got your hopes up. This exercise is an extension of the earlier wall roll-up that allows you to safely move into hyperextension of the back, targeting the back extensors and deep posterior muscles again, along with the hip extensors (the butt muscles) and upper-back muscles. A lot of people I've trained had a hard time with this exercise in the beginning because it really makes you stretch out and into a position that you don't normally get into. The reason for adding an exercise like this is that it teaches you to contract and hold the back and glute muscles, which gives your posture a boost and helps balance the strength of the abdominal muscles and hip flexors.

Preparation

1. Lie face down on the floor on either an exercise mat or a carpeted surface.

2. Stretch your arms out over your head and point your toes, but keep everything on the floor. This should look like Superman flying.

Movement

3. Move into the first position by lifting your head, arms, and shoulders off the floor as far as possible. Don't push against the floor with your hands; your back muscles have to do all the work. You will probably be able to lift your chest only an inch or two off the floor, at most.

4. Move into the second position by lifting both legs off the floor as high as possible. Keep your legs straight, and really concentrate on using your back and butt muscles to lift. You should really feel this in your back (that's a good feeling). Hold this position for up to 60 seconds.

5. Relax back to the floor and rest for 15–20 seconds before doing another repetition. Your goal should be to do five repetitions of 60 seconds without any effort.

Precautions

If you feel any pain in your back during this exercise, or if your back muscles start to cramp, stop and relax. This exercise may be too advanced for you right now. Talk with your doctor before you try it again.

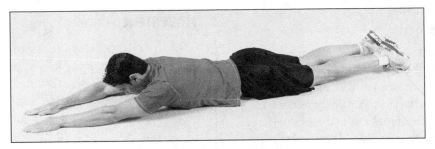

Starting/ending position.

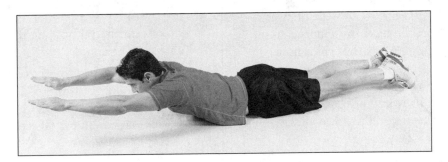

First position.

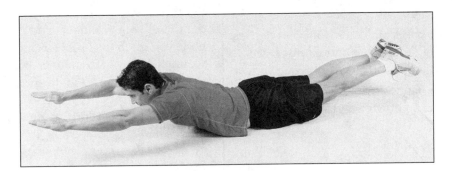

Second position.

Bridging

Bridging is an exercise that targets the hip extensor muscles of your glutes for movement, and your back extensors and deep posterior muscles for stabilization. You may also feel your thigh muscles working because you have to push on your feet, which makes your legs want to straighten out. This is another stretch that a lot of new clients struggle with in the beginning. I think it has to do with the weakness that most people have in their back muscles, so we are going to fix that right now. After just a few sessions with this exercise, you will notice a serious improvement in the strength of your back and how easy it is to sit up straight and keep good posture all day long.

Preparation

1. Lie down on your back on a carpeted surface, or use an exercise mat.

2. Bend your knees and keep your feet flat on the floor. Your heels should be placed no more than a foot away from your butt.

3. Place both hands down at your sides, palms pressing down against the floor.

Movement

4. In one smooth motion, lift your hips into the air until your knees, hips, and shoulders are in a straight line. Do not lift your hips to the point that you can't see your knees. You can push against the floor with your hands to help lift your hips, if you need to. With practice and increasing strength, your back and hip muscles will do all the work.

5. Concentrate on holding this position for up to 60 seconds.

6. Slowly relax and lower your hips back to the ground. Rest for 15–20 seconds and do another repetition. A goal of 10 repetitions, each held for 60 seconds, is ideal.

Precautions

Because you are supporting a lot of weight on the top of your shoulders and the base of your neck, you might feel some strain in these areas. If so, immediately relax and rest before attempting another repetition. If you experience any pain in your neck from this exercise, stop and consult with your doctor before attempting it again.

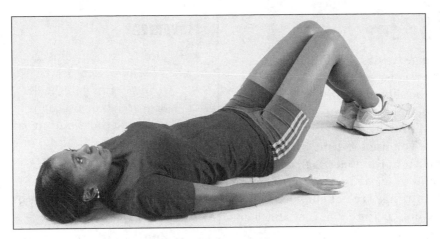

Starting/ending position.

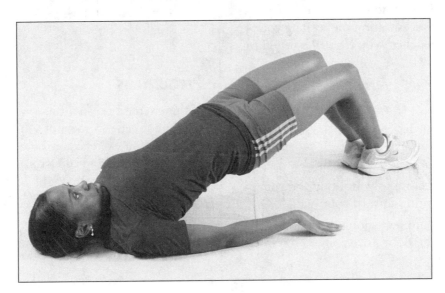

Midpoint position.

Straight Bridge

The straight bridge exercise is a little more demanding than regular bridging. It is deceiving because you are not lifting your body as high off the floor, but a lot of different muscles are involved that you normally don't use all at the same time. Here you use the same back extensors and deep posterior muscles as in regular bridging, but now you also involve your hamstrings. The hamstrings are not considered part of the core musculature, but they attach at the hip and help to extend your hip, so they will become involved in this exercise—and you will definitely feel it! Additionally, if you focus some of your concentration on keeping your butt muscles clenched, you'll get the benefit of a tighter butt.

Preparation

1. Lie on your back on an exercise mat or carpeted surface.

2. Prop yourself up on your elbows, keeping your arms close to your body and your hands pointing toward your feet.

3. Your legs and feet should be together, heels on the floor, toes pointed toward the ceiling.

Movement

4. Slowly lift your hips, contracting the muscles of your lower back and hamstrings, until your heels, hips, and shoulders are all in a straight line (don't forget to clench those butt muscles). This requires you to lift up only about 6–8 inches, so it's not a very big movement.

5. Hold this position for up to 60 seconds, or until you start to sag back toward the ground when the muscles get fatigued.

6. Rest 15–20 seconds before your next repetition. Keep at this exercise until you can complete 10 repetitions of 60 seconds each.

Precautions

If this exercise is too difficult to maintain position for at least 15 seconds, go back to the regular bridging exercise until the lower-back and glute muscles are a little stronger. Also, if you feel any pain or cramping in your back, stop and consult with your doctor before attempting this exercise again.

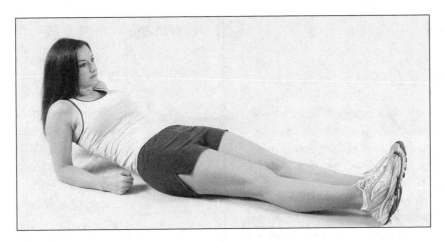

Starting/ending position.

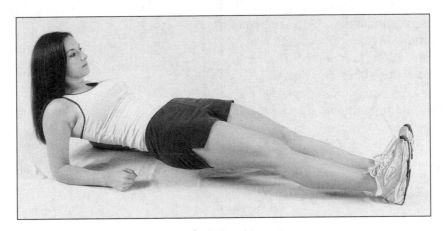

Midpoint position.

Side Bend

Side bends have been around forever, but very few people actually do them anymore. That's about to change because side bends are an excellent core-conditioning exercise that gets both your abdominal and lower-back muscles working together. In this exercise, you move laterally, or to the sides, rather than to the front and back. This allows muscles that normally oppose each other to work with each other, giving you another level of core strength and stability. You will notice the benefits of this exercise any time you have to carry something heavy, such as a suitcase, in one hand without anything in the opposite hand to help keep you balanced and upright. Again, only gravity is at work, so there isn't a lot of resistance. Side bends are really a postural exercise that is designed to help keep you standing upright, straight, and tall, and prepare you for more difficult exercises later.

Preparation

1. Stand with your feet together, arms at your sides.
2. If you are a little unsteady in this position, keep your feet a couple of inches apart.

Movement

3. Slowly lean to one side, running your hand down the side of your leg as far as you can go without losing your balance.
4. Return to the upright position and lean to the other side as far as you can.
5. Keep your hand against the side of your body at all times. This will ensure that you are bending to the side, not forward or backward.
6. This exercise is not taxing, so concentrate on reaching down as far as you can. When you can get your hand past your knee, you'll know you're in good shape.

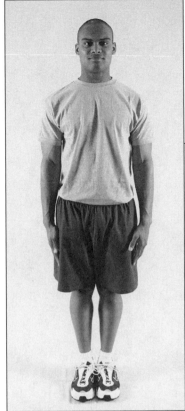

Starting/ending position.

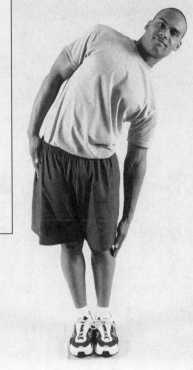

Left midpoint position.

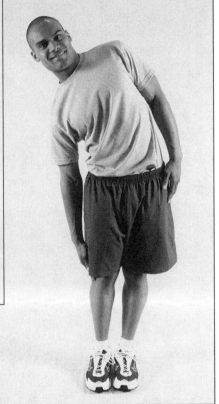

Right midpoint position.

In This Chapter

◆ Gravity gets stronger

◆ Moving multiple muscles together

◆ Adding rotation and balance

◆ Exercises with a twist

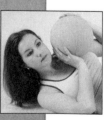
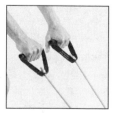
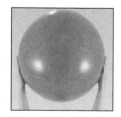
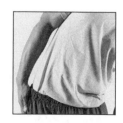
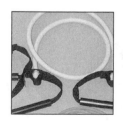
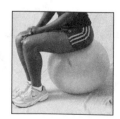

Chapter 5

Advanced Body Weight Exercises

When you have mastered the beginning body weighted exercises, you can move on to these more advanced movements. It's important that you really get good at the beginning moves before you go much further because you want to establish a solid foundation to build upon, and certainly prevent any injuries.

This chapter pushes you further than you probably ever thought you could go without using exercise equipment. Gravity is still acting as the resistance, but now you will put your body into positions that make you use several muscle groups at the same time to achieve the goal. This makes the exercises more effective at training your core muscles and really gives you that feeling that you are getting stronger (and more tired) with every move. I introduce you to exercises that involve balance, rotation, and coordination (no more just standing still). If you're one of those people who think they have two left feet, keep working hard and you'll be able to conquer these exercises with practice and determination—and then hit that dance floor and be graceful.

Cycling

For this exercise, you use an imaginary bicycle (and wear an imaginary helmet, just in case you crash). Because the bike is pretend, this type of cycling is actually a core-conditioning exercise that targets both the hip extensors and hip flexors for movement, while your lower-back muscles provide stabilization. This takes some practice because you will be moving in the same pattern as if you were riding a bike, but without any of the resistance of actual pedals. What makes this exercise different and effective is that you have to learn to control the movement of your legs in space without any resistance other than gravity. It sounds easy, and it will be once you get the hang of it, but if you feel a little unsteady in the beginning, that's okay—you're normal, and you don't have far to fall.

Preparation

1. Lie on your back on an exercise mat or carpeted surface.

2. Prop yourself up on your elbows, keeping your arms close to your body and your hands pointing toward your feet.

3. Lift both legs up in the air, pointing your left leg straight out away from you, and bring the right knee up close to you.

Movement

4. Pretend you are riding a bike, moving your feet in a circular motion. Each time you bring a leg up, bend the knee as much as you can, really bringing it up close to your chest. Each time you straighten a leg, point your toe and completely flatten your knee.

5. Never let your feet touch the ground, and don't lift them any higher than your head. Continue rotating in a circular motion for up to 60 seconds.

6. Relax and rest for 15–20 seconds before your next repetition. For variety, you can alternate the direction of your rotations forward and backward with each set. Complete two sets forward and two sets backward (each of them 60 seconds long), and you'll be ready to hit the road.

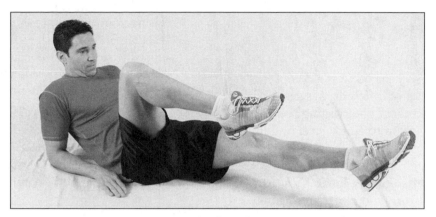

Starting/ending position.

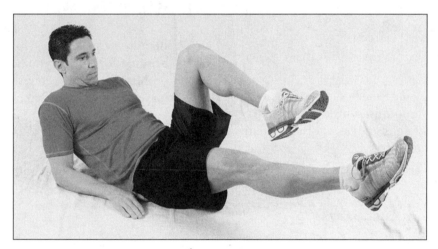

Midpoint position.

Twisting Toe Touch

Rotation is a motion that looks really easy on the outside but, to your body, is a complex interaction of a lot of different muscles that have to work together. The twisting toe touch exercise takes rotation to a new level by adding a forward bend at the hip at the same time (technically called hip-flexion). Here you will be working the abdominals, lower back, back extensors, hip flexors, and glutes all together. This is a real multimuscle exercise that will get your blood flowing and that's great for loosening up a stiff back first thing in the morning or after a long day at work.

Preparation

1. Stand with your feet shoulder-width apart, toes pointed out just a little bit. Keep your legs straight and do not move them during the exercise.
2. Hold your arms out to each side at shoulder level.

Movement

3. Starting with either arm, bend over and touch the opposite toe. The left hand reaches over and touches the right toe, or the right hand reaches over and touches the left toe. The other hand reaches up in the air above you. Be sure to breathe out as you go down.

4. Using your back and glute muscles, stand back up and repeat the toe touch to the opposite side. Breathe back in as you stand up. Alternate side to side until you have completed all your repetitions (about 20 reps in a set is good).
5. Make sure you stand all the way back up before you start the next repetition. It's cheating if you don't get all the way back to the starting point before the next repetition.

Precautions

◆ Because this exercise involves rotation and bending forward, if you have any back problems, you probably shouldn't attempt it. See your doctor if you aren't sure.

◆ Don't go too fast during this exercise. Moving your head up and down like this can cause dizziness. If you feel dizzy or lightheaded, sit down and rest until this goes away. Then the next time you do this exercise, slow down and take deep breaths.

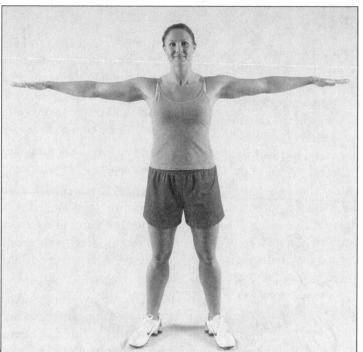

Starting/ending position.

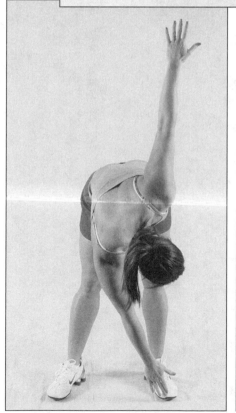

Left side midpoint position.

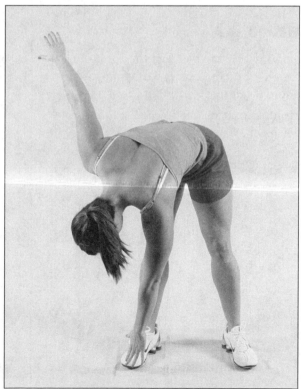

Right side midpoint position.

Balanced Toe Touch

This exercise takes the twisting toe touch to an even higher level, so make sure you are comfortable and good at doing that exercise first. We already have rotation, flexion, and extension covered, so we're now going to add the dimension of balance to push you a little bit more. Any time you have to balance and move at the same time, gravity gets an advantage over you—and tries to knock you down. When you have less contact with the ground (standing on one foot instead of two), the muscles in one leg have to hold up all your body weight instead of dividing it between both legs. This means that you have to work even harder to coordinate the muscles you are using to get the job done. Practice this exercise slowly at first until you get the feel for it; then you can add a little more speed to your movements and really engage those core muscles.

Preparation

1. Stand with your feet together or just a couple of inches apart, with your toes pointed out just a little bit.
2. Hold your arms out to each side at shoulder level.

Movement

3. Lift your right leg to balance on your left. At the same time, reach down with your right hand and touch your left toe. As you reach down, let your right leg move out behind you and your left arm move up in the air to help with balance.
4. Using your back and glute muscles, stand back up and put your right foot back down.
5. Repeat to the opposite side by balancing on your right leg and reaching down with your left hand to touch your right toe. Alternate side to side until you have completed all your repetitions (three sets of 20 reps is pretty good).
6. Make sure you stand all the way back up before you start the next repetition. It's cheating if you don't get all the way back to the starting point before the next repetition.

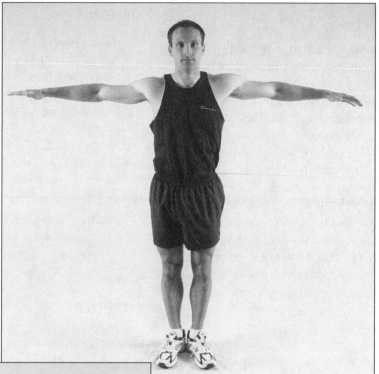

Starting/ending position.

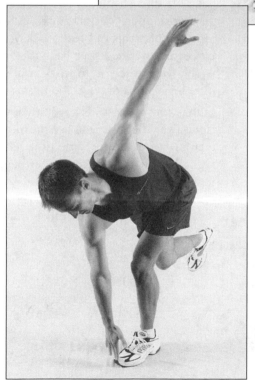

Left midpoint position.

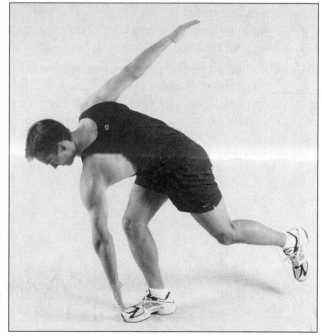

Right midpoint position.

Double Crunch

If you want to really get all your abdominal muscles working together, look no further than the double crunch. Because you are combining elements of the abdominal crunch and reverse crunch at the same time, this "doubles" the level of difficulty. On top of this, because both your shoulder and your hips will be leaving the floor at the same time, you have to balance your body on just the middle of your back without falling over to the side. The double crunch is a highly efficient exercise because you're working the entire abdominal muscle—upper and lower—with one exercise. When you do it correctly, you will feel the burn throughout the abs (and you'll probably be calling me names, too).

Preparation

1. Lie down on your back on a carpeted surface, or use an exercise mat.

2. Hold your legs straight up in the air without lifting your hips off the floor. Pretend you are putting your feet on the ceiling (like your mother told you never to do).

3. Put your arms straight up in the air, too. During the movement, you are going to try to touch your toes, so aim your fingers now.

Movement

4. Take a deep breath in. As you blow it out, roll your shoulders up until the shoulder blades leave the floor, and roll your hips up until your butt is off the floor. Crunch from both ends at the same time, pushing your feet toward the ceiling and trying to touch your toes with your hands. The only thing left touching the floor should be your lower and middle back.

5. Slowly unroll yourself back to the starting position, and keep repeating until you can't touch your toes anymore or you get to 40 reps—which is plenty of this exercise.

Precautions

◆ Perform this exercise slowly and take very deep breaths. If you get tired and start getting sloppy by jerking or trying to use momentum, stop and rest. Lack of control can cause the lower back to contract, which will cause you to work your back muscles instead of your abdominals.

◆ Don't worry if you can't reach your toes right away. Because you are pushing your feet farther up at the same time, you really have to crunch the upper part of your body to reach. As your core gets stronger, the movement will become easier and you'll be able to fully crunch.

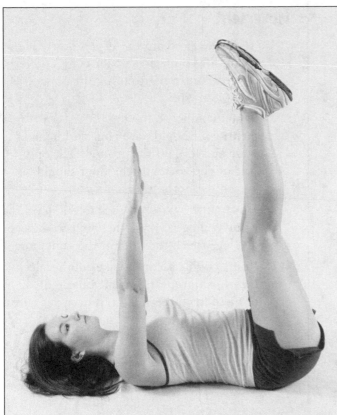

Starting/ending position.

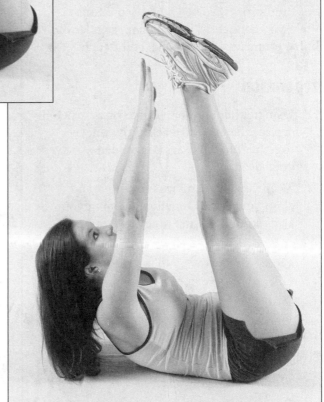

Midpoint position.

V-Up

The V-up was given its name because when you look at this from the side, you are forming the letter *V*. This exercise takes the double crunch and adds more intensity by having you start with your arms and legs extended from your body. This gives gravity another advantage. The farther out you extend your arms and legs from your core, the harder your core muscles have to work to bring them back together. When you do this exercise, you also have that pesky balance to deal with again (funny how that keeps popping up, almost as if I'd planned it). The V-up takes some practice to get right and to do very many repetitions. It's an intense exercise that makes all your abdominal muscles work together and gets your hip flexors involved at the same time. When you conquer this challenge, regular old double crunches will look like child's play.

Preparation

1. Using either an exercise mat or a carpeted surface, lie on your back with your feet together and your arms extended out over your head.

2. Keep your feet and legs together, and clasp your hands together, keeping your arms straight all the time.

Movement

3. Take a deep breath in. As you slowly blow it out, lift your arms, upper body, and legs into the air, trying to bring them together over your hips.

4. When you get to the top of the movement, you should have your entire upper body and legs off the ground. The only part of you touching the floor should be your hips and butt.

5. Slowly lower yourself back to the floor. Time your descent so that your shoulders and legs touch the floor at the same time.

6. Rest a couple seconds, take another deep breath, and repeat. When you can do 40 of these for three sets, consider your core fully worked.

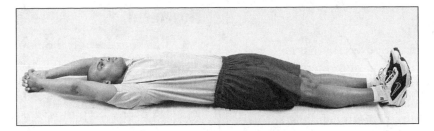

Starting/ending position.

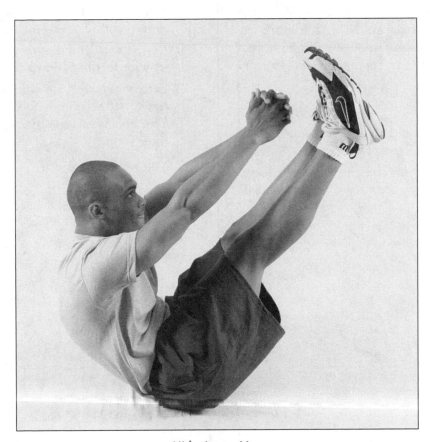

Midpoint position.

Tuck

Tucks are a new kind of exercise that involves balance, stabilization, and movement all at the same time. This is a heftier challenge for your abdominals and hip flexors than they've seen before—but I'm sure you can handle it at this point. This is one of those exercises that you will grow to both love and hate. It really makes the abdominal muscles scream because they don't get a chance to rest during the entire set. Although your posture will thank you for it, your brain will probably be calling me names again.

Preparation

1. Sit upright on the floor with your feet extended in front of you.

2. Hold your arms straight out at shoulder level, and keep them there the whole time.

Movement

3. Lift your feet off the floor and bring your knees up toward your chest. You may feel yourself leaning back a little bit to stay balanced. That's fine as long as you don't fall over—keep those abs tight!

4. Extend your legs back out straight, but don't let them touch the floor. As soon as they are straight, bring your knees back up toward your chest to the tucked position.

5. Repeat until your entire set is done; then let your feet back down to the floor.

6. Let your abs rest a moment. Lie back and rest 15–20 seconds before your next set. Your goal is 40 repetitions per set for three sets.

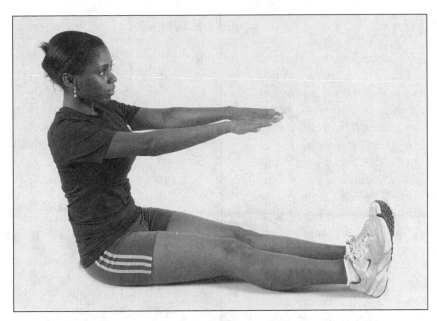

Starting/ending position.

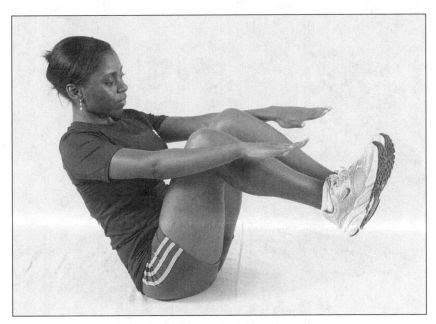

Midpoint position.

Balanced Twist

Here we go with the balance again—but this time with a twist. This movement should be done very slowly so you can concentrate on letting your core muscles move and coordinate the balance. You won't really feel this exercise burn as much as the others; it's more about control and coordination. The focus here is on the range of motion you can achieve while standing on one foot—you'll see that one direction will be easier than the other—so really push yourself where it's hardest, and you'll see the benefits later during more difficult exercises.

Preparation

1. Stand with your feet together, arms held out in front of you, hands clasped together.

Movement

2. Lift one foot off the ground and get balanced before you start moving.

3. Slowly rotate your body in the direction opposite of the leg you are standing on. Twist yourself as far around as you can while keeping your arms held out straight.

4. Slowly move back toward the other side, twisting to the same side as the leg you are standing on. Go as far in this direction as you can while keeping your arms held out straight.

5. Repeat 10 twists to each side for one set; then rest for a minute and switch legs for another set.

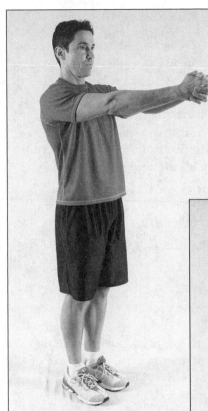

Starting/ending position.

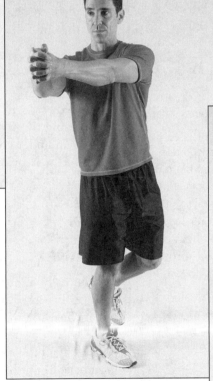

Opposite side midpoint position.

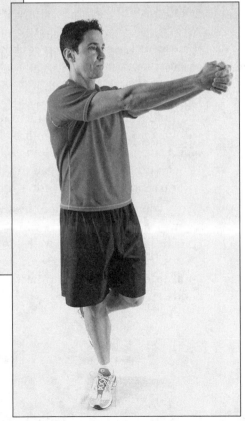

Same side midpoint position.

Modified Sit-Up

Now we take the ordinary sit-up (see Chapter 4) that you are probably getting sick of by now and make it a little harder by taking away an anchor point. By having only one leg on the ground, the hip flexors of that leg have to work even harder (actually twice as hard and twice the fun). Doing this is similar to balancing, except that it is hard to stand up and do a sit-up. When you make one side of your body work harder than the other, the core muscles have to adapt to keep you from falling over to one side. You'll definitely notice the difference when you do these, and your friends will be impressed with your new skills.

Preparation

1. Lie down on your back on a carpeted surface, or use an exercise mat.

2. Bend your knees and keep your feet flat on the floor. Your heels should be placed no more than a foot away from your butt. Choose which leg you want to start with, and hold it up in the air. The other leg will have to be anchored under a heavy object, or have someone hold your foot. When you get stronger, you can do this without anchoring your foot.

3. Cross your arms over your chest. If you want to put your hands on the side of your head, that's okay as well. However, do not lock your hands together under your head or support your head with your hands.

Movement

4. Take a deep breath in. As you blow it out, roll your head and shoulders off the ground toward your knees (this is basically an abdominal crunch so far). When your shoulders leave the floor, keep your abdominals contracted and begin pulling with the hip flexor muscles to bring your entire back all the way off the floor.

5. Touch your elbow to your knee, and slowly lower yourself back to the floor.

6. Repeat for one set, rest, and then complete another set with the opposite leg in the air.

Precautions

When you start to get tired, concentrate on performing the abdominal crunch portion of the sit-up under control. Do not let yourself get into the habit of jerking up off the floor when your abs get tired. This will cause the back muscles to contract and could cause injury.

Variations

If you really want to impress those around you, and really want a challenging sit-up, don't use an anchor. You may have to move your foot a little farther away from you, but it will really engage the hip flexors on that side and make you have to put in some real effort.

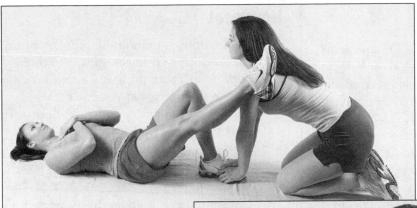

Starting/ending position.

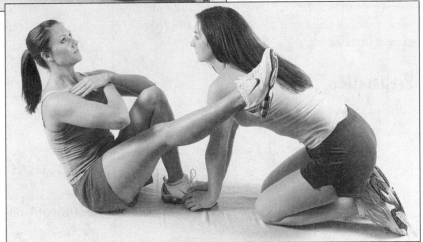

Midpoint position.

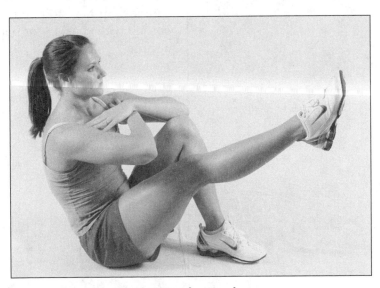

Variation without anchor.

Modified Bridging

A modified bridge uses the same concept as the modified sit-up: only one leg to work with. If you do modified sit-ups, you'll want to do modified bridging because they work opposing muscle groups (abs and hip flexors vs. lower back and hip extensors). In this exercise, your lowerback, deep posterior, and glute muscles will be doing all the work. As before, because you will be touching the floor with only one leg, the side you use will be working harder, and your core muscles will have to coordinate and balance a little more.

Preparation

1. Lie down on your back on a carpeted surface, or use an exercise mat.

2. Bend your knees and keep your feet flat on the floor. Your heels should be placed no more than a foot away from your butt. Lift one leg off the floor and hold it straight out.

3. Place both hands down at your sides, palms pressing down against the floor.

Movement

4. In one smooth motion, lift your hips into the air until your knees, hips, and shoulders are in a straight line. Do not lift your hips to the point that you can't see your knees. You can push against the floor with your hands to help lift your hips, if you need to. With practice and increasing strength, your back and hip muscles will do all the work.

5. Concentrate on holding this position for up to 60 seconds.

6. Slowly relax and lower your hips back to the ground. Rest for 15–20 seconds and repeat with the other leg in the air. Repeat by alternating which leg is held in the air. Two sets on each leg should be plenty.

Precautions

Because you are supporting a lot of weight on the top of your shoulders and the base of your neck, you might feel some strain in these areas. If so, immediately relax and rest before attempting another repetition. If you experience any pain in your neck from this exercise, stop and consult with your doctor before attempting it again.

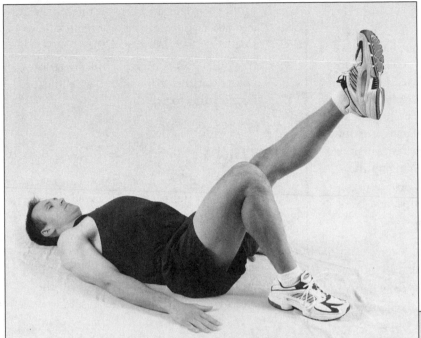

Starting/ending position.

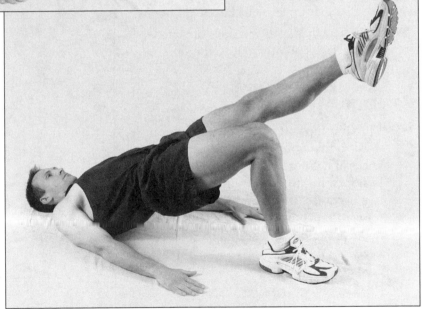

Midpoint position.

Kneeling Twist

A kneeling twist is an exercise that has a lot of variability that you can adjust to make it more difficult. This is one body weighted exercise that you probably won't ever outgrow—you can just keep making it harder (yea!). This exercise combines elements of balance, rotation, and speed. You can do several different versions of this exercise in one workout, changing the angle and speed to vary the intensity, and getting more of your abdominals, hips, and back muscles involved as you choose.

Preparation

1. Kneel on the floor, keeping your feet and knees together, and sitting back on your heels. You'll probably want to use an exercise mat under your knees.

2. Hold your hands to the sides of your head, elbows pointed out to the sides.

Movement

3. Lift your hips off your feet, and lean forward so that your chest is in front of your knees. The more you lift your hips and lean forward, the more difficult this exercise becomes. If you find that leaning forward on your knees hurts or is too difficult right now, stay seated back on your heels.

4. Hold your legs and hips in one position, and twist your upper body from side to side as far as you can.

5. As you are able, increase the speed of your rotations from side to side and/or lean farther forward.

Precautions

Focus on the range of motion you can reach before you start increasing the speed. When you do start going faster, be careful of the "bounce" at the end of a rotation when changing directions. The idea is to make your muscles work, but too much stretch at the end of a rotation could cause an injury. Control the speed, and you control the muscles.

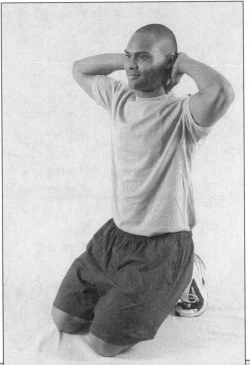

Starting/ending position.

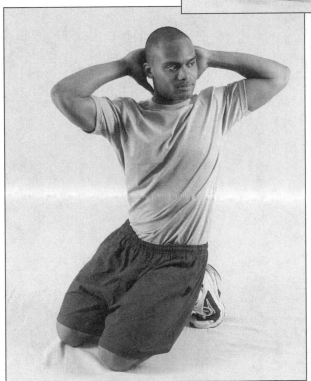

Midpoint position on your heels.

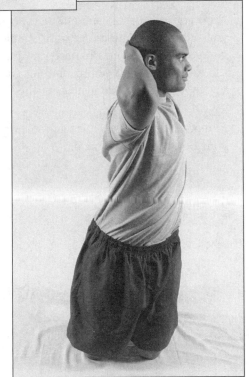

Midpoint position leaning forward.

Side Bridge

The side bridge takes the movement of the side bend (see Chapter 4) and makes it a little harder. As with the side bend, the abdominal and lower-back muscles will be working together, but this time they will be working to stabilize and move your body. Additionally, your muscles of your upper back will be working to stabilize the shoulder you will be leaning against, and your glutes will be working to lift your hips up in the air. All the muscles working together on this one is sure to make your core stronger.

Preparation

1. Lie on the floor on your side, with one leg on top of the other. It doesn't matter which side; you'll be doing both before it's over.

2. Prop yourself up on one elbow. Keep your elbow directly under your shoulder, and your forearm and hand flat against the ground. At this point, none of your upper body should be touching the floor except that arm.

3. Extend the arm that is not supporting your body over your head.

Movement

4. Lift your hips off the ground until your body is in a straight line. Hold this position for up to 60 seconds.

5. Relax back to the floor, roll over to the other side, and complete another repetition.

6. Continue alternating side bridges on each side until you have completed three sets on each side.

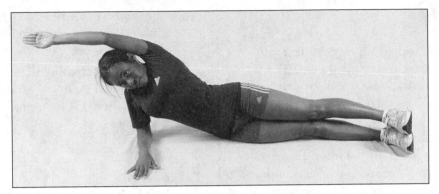

Starting/ending position.

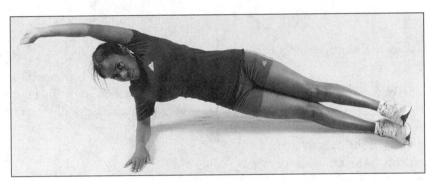

Midpoint position.

Windmill

Windmills are another old exercise that you used to see a lot on the football field. It's a good exercise for loosening up your entire core, and it involves rotation while bent over. This makes gravity work to try to push you all the way over, while your core muscles work to keep you moving and off the floor. Done correctly, this is a great exercise that uses both the abdominal and back muscles for rotation, and the hips and hamstrings to keep you stable.

Preparation

1. Stand with your feet slightly wider than shoulder-width apart.
2. Hold your arms straight out to your sides.
3. Bend at the waist until your legs and upper body are at a 90-degree angle. If you can't get this far over, just go as far as you can, but not beyond 90 degrees.

Movement

4. Keeping your arms straight out to your sides, rotate your upper body so that one arm moves toward the floor and the other toward the ceiling. Rotate as far as you can under control.

5. When you have rotated as far as you can, change directions and go back the other way as far as you can.
6. Continue alternating directions until you have rotated each way 10 times. That's one set. Rest 15–20 seconds and complete two more sets.

Precautions

◆ Be careful not to move too fast on this one. Speed is not an issue here, so move slowly and deliberately, letting your muscles do the work.

◆ If you feel dizzy or lightheaded at any time, stop and sit down. You were probably just holding your breath. Remember to breathe naturally during this exercise.

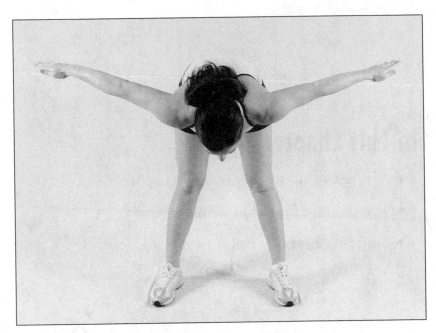

Starting/ending position.

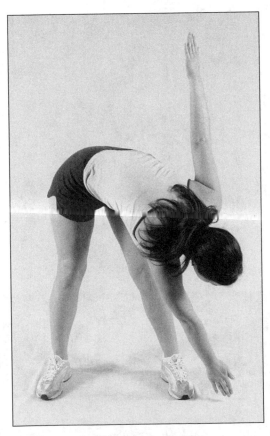

Left side midpoint position.

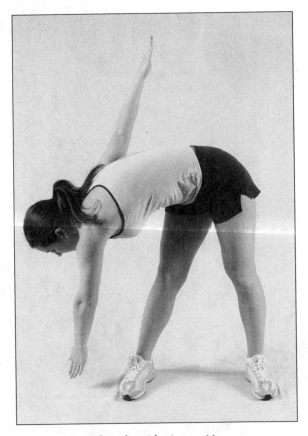

Right side midpoint position.

In This Chapter

- ◆ Using tubing to challenge your core
- ◆ Punching, crunching, and chopping
- ◆ Building on body weight exercises
- ◆ Kneeling for more power

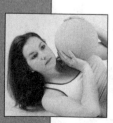
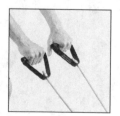
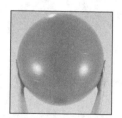
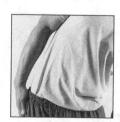
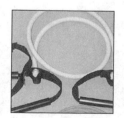
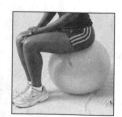

Chapter 6

Beginning Resistance Tubing Exercises

Ever take a rubber band and see how far you could stretch it? I have, and if you have, too, you know that it gets harder and harder to stretch, until it pops and stings your hand. Somewhere down the road, some bright person thought it would be a good idea to make really big rubber bands with handles on the end, and then use them to exercise their muscles. That was one smart person. We should thank them for inventing what we now call resistance tubing because it gives us a whole new way to challenge our core muscles.

This chapter moves you beyond body weight exercises, adding resistance tubing to enhance the effect of gravity and allow us to work in different directions. From here on out, the exercises just keep on getting better. In my humble opinion, resistance tubing has peanut butter and jelly sandwiches beat hands down as one of the greatest inventions in history. Although you can't eat it, resistance tubing opens up so many possibilities and can be used in so many ways that entire books have been dedicated to the subject. I've picked the best ones to test your core muscles and push your core-conditioning program. Now it's just up to you to do the work—I'm going to go eat a peanut butter and jelly sandwich.

Twisting Punch

The twisting punch is an exercise that originated on the mean streets of Inmymind as a fighting technique. Actually, I just made that up, but it sounds cool, right? The twisting punch is not a fighting move or a spiked drink; it's a very controlled rotational movement that engages the muscles of your core to provide stability and action. In this exercise, you use your abdominals, back muscles, hip rotators, and shoulder stabilizers all at the same time. This exercise won't turn you into Bruce Lee, but he would probably agree this is a great exercise. You don't have to do this punch quickly, but after you master the technique, adding speed will help you produce power. All of my clients love this exercise because it also teaches them to control the nondominant side of their body just as well as their dominant side.

Preparation

1. Attach one end of your resistance tube to your door-jamb anchor or around a pole at shoulder height. Hold the other end in one hand. If you want to double the resistance, loop your tubing so you are holding both handles in one hand.

2. Hold the tubing in one hand close to your shoulder, and keep your elbow bent and next to your body. Your other hand should be on your hip. Face away from the tubing anchor point.

3. Move away from the anchor point until all the slack is out of the tubing. Stand with your feet shoulder-width apart. The foot on the same side as the hand holding the tubing should be slightly in front of the other foot, for a good, stable base.

Movement

4. The exercise is a combination of rotation and extension of your arm. The arm movement is not a part of the core conditioning, but it gives you a focus point for the movement.

5. Start pushing your hand away from your body, pretending you are punching someone in front of you in slow motion. At the same time, start rotating your body so that the hand with the tubing in it can reach as far in front of you as possible.

6. Completely rotate your body as far as you can, pushing out on the tubing. When you get to the end of the rotation, slowly return to the starting point, bringing your hand back to your shoulder and twisting back the way you came.

7. Repeat the motion for one set; then switch sides and work the other arm and direction of rotation.

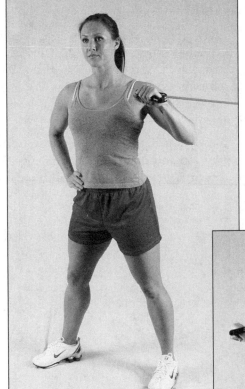

Starting/ending position.

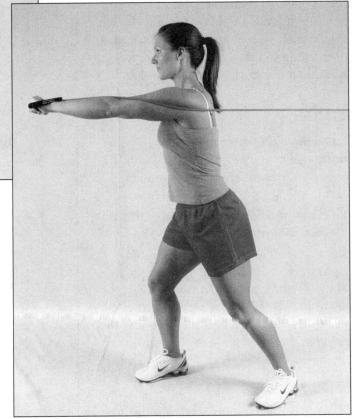

Midpoint position.

Overhead Crunch

The overhead crunch allows you to add resistance to an abdominal exercise. You can use as heavy a resistance tube as you can handle (you'll be able to handle more than you think). As with the abdominal crunch you do on the floor (see Chapter 4), this exercise targets the big surface muscle (the rectus abdominis) and the obliques deep inside. A lot of my clients use this exercise simply because the regular abdominal crunch becomes boring when you have to do 100 of them just to start feeling it. If you aren't to that point yet, you'll get there really soon and you'll be happy that there is a way to make the crunch harder (although your friends may look at you funny for trying to make crunches harder, you'll be the one with the strong core).

Preparation

1. Loop your resistance tube through your door anchor or over the top of a pole above your head. Hold one handle in each hand.

2. Kneel on the floor directly under the tubing. Sit back on your heels.

3. Bend your elbows and hold the tubing right next to each shoulder. Keep your elbows tight against your body. There shouldn't be any slack in the tubing at this point—if there is, adjust it by looping the tubing around the pole or through the anchor again.

Movement

4. Starting in an upright position, slowly crunch down so your head moves toward your knees. You won't go all the way to your knees, just into a fetal position, allowing the abdominal muscles to flex you forward.

5. Slowly unroll yourself back to an upright position and repeat the movement. Three sets of 30 reps is a good goal to start with.

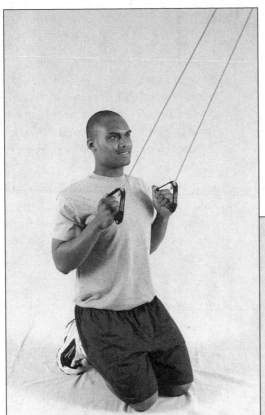

Starting/ending position.

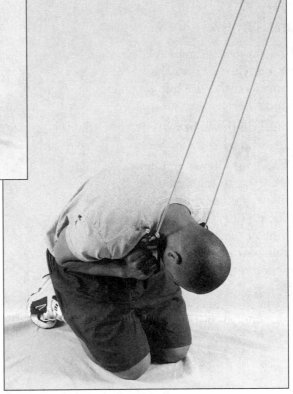

Midpoint position.

Overhead Oblique

The overhead oblique exercise is almost exactly like the overhead crunch, except that you are going to add some rotation as you flex downward. This allows the obliques to engage more during the movement, and gets more of the deeper core muscles involved. The tubing will really stretch out as you rotate, and one side will feel like it's pulling more than the other—that's normal. Work on this exercise until you can do three sets of 30 reps. By then, your abs will be asking for a break.

Preparation

1. Loop your resistance tube through your door anchor or over the top of a pole above your head. Hold one handle in each hand.

2. Kneel on the floor directly under the tubing. Sit back on your heels.

3. Bend your elbows and hold the tubing right next to each shoulder. Keep your elbows tight against your body. There shouldn't be any slack in the tubing at this point. If there is, adjust it by looping the tubing around the pole or through the anchor again.

Movement

4. Starting in an upright position, slowly crunch over, bringing your head down toward your knees. As you flex downward, rotate your shoulders so that during one repetition, your right shoulder crosses over toward your left knee, and on the next repetition, your left shoulder crosses over toward your right knee.

5. Slowly unroll yourself back to an upright position and repeat the movement to the other side. Alternate left and right rotations to complete the set.

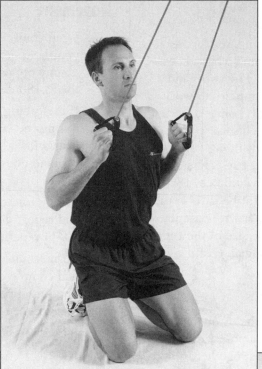

Starting/ending position.

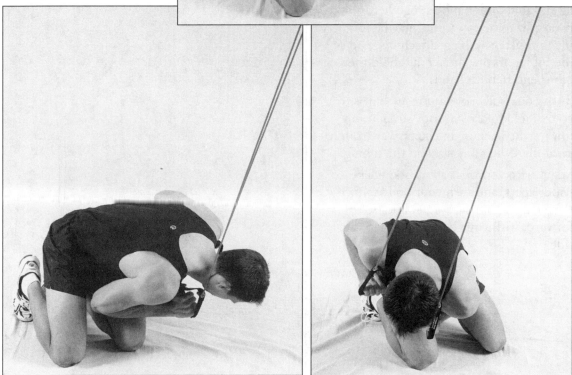

Left midpoint position.   Right midpoint position.

Two-Hand Twist

When you use resistance tubing, the farther it stretches and moves away from your core, the harder the exercise becomes. The two-hand twist really forces your core muscles to work because the resistance tubing is going to stretch a long way from your body. This exercise involves all the core muscles, including your shoulder stabilizers and upper back. The goal of this exercise is to achieve a complete 180 degrees of rotation. This might be hard in the beginning, but it will get easier with practice, and then you can increase the size of the resistance tube and make it hard again (yea!).

Preparation

1. Loop your resistance tube through your door anchor or around a pole at shoulder level. Hold both handles together in both hands. In some cases, this may be too much resistance. If so, attach one end of the tubing to the anchor and hold the other end in both hands.

2. Turn your body so that the anchor is to your side. Hold your arms straight out toward the anchor, and step away from it until there isn't any slack in the tubing.

3. Stand with your feet about shoulder-width apart, and turn your body to face the anchor. Your feet should be facing forward, with your body rotated to one side.

Movement

4. Keep your arms straight. Slowly rotate your body until your arms are pointing exactly opposite from where they started; this is 180 degrees.

5. If the tubing touches your chest or arms during the last part of the rotation, step back a little bit so it is more in front of you and doesn't interfere with your movement.

6. Slowly rotate back to the starting point and repeat until you have finished a set of 10–15 repetitions.

7. Turn around to face the other direction and complete another set, rotating the opposite direction from the first set (left to right, or right to left). Complete four total sets (two on each side).

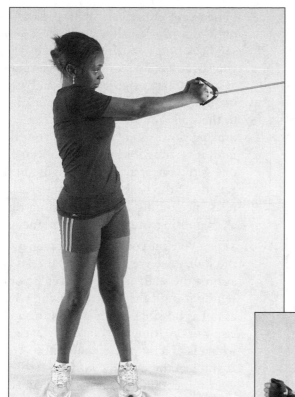

Starting/ending position.

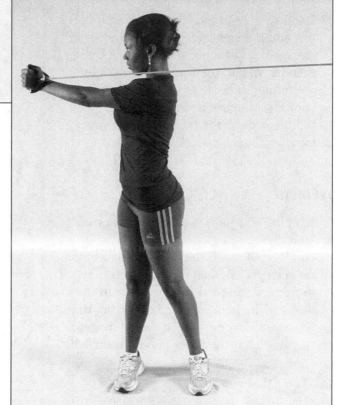

Midpoint position.

Resisted Wall Roll-Up

This exercise targets the muscles that perform exactly opposite of the abdominal muscles, and it is the partner exercise to the overhead crunch and overhead obliques. The back extensors (erector spinae and deep posterior muscles) work during this exercise to take you from a bent-over position to a standing position. The resistance tubing and our old friend gravity will be attempting to pull you back down toward the ground, so these core muscles have to work hard to get the job done.

Preparation

1. Stand with your back against a wall and your feet about a foot in front of you.

2. Loop your resistance tubing under both feet and hold a handle in each hand. Your arms will stay at your sides for this entire exercise. Make sure there is no slack in the tubing. If there is, you can spread your feet wider to make the tubing tighter, or loop the tubing around your feet.

Movement

3. Keeping your hips against the wall, tuck your chin to your chest and slowly roll your vertebrae off the wall, one at a time. To keep you focused on the correct movement, pretend you are stuck to the wall and are being "peeled off" from the top down. The resistance should be getting lighter as the tubing is less stretched.

4. When your entire back is off the wall and only your hips remain, slowly raise yourself back to the starting position by rolling your back against the wall one vertebrae at a time, starting at your hips and working up. Think of this as being stuck back to the wall. You want to concentrate on moving slowly and "unrolling" your body until it is straight again. The movement of one vertebrae at a time will highlight the activity of the back extensor muscles. The resistance tubing should be getting tighter and opposing your upward movement.

5. When you get your entire back against the wall, raise your head until it rests against the wall, and try to stretch yourself up toward the ceiling, making yourself as tall as possible. You may feel this exercise working only in your lower back, which is exactly where you want to feel it. If you feel the muscles working farther up your spine, that just means those muscles needed some more work and are getting stronger as well.

6. Relax your back and begin another repetition. Finish three sets of 10–15 reps, and your back will be one of the strongest on the block.

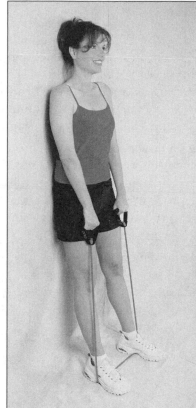

Starting/ending position.

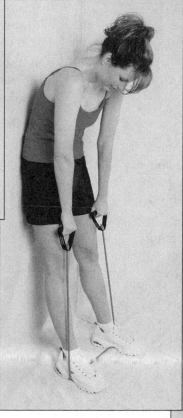

Halfway up position.

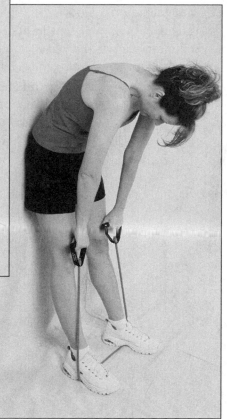

Midpoint position.

Stump Puller

I doubt you will ever actually need this exercise to get ready to pull a real tree stump out of the ground, but you never know. Actually, the movement is so named because it mimics the movement that you would perform to pull something heavy out of the ground. The core muscles of the back and shoulders are the main workers in this exercise. Your lower-back muscles provide all the stabilization and will be working the whole time as well. Another neat thing about this exercise is that it has an element of power that will really get your core firing fast and strong. Have fun, and remember that trees are your friends.

Preparation

1. Attach your resistance tubing through your door anchor at foot level or under something heavy, such as a leg of your couch. Hold one handle in each hand.

2. Stand up straight, hold your hands down in front of you, and step back until there isn't any slack in the tubing.

3. Slightly bend your knees and hips.

Movement

4. With a quick, powerful movement, lift your arms in the air over your head, and extend your knees and hips so you are reaching as high as you can. Don't bend your arms; keep them straight at all times.

5. The stretch of the resistance tubing will be pulling you back down, and this is one case in which you won't fight it. As soon as you get your hands over your head, let them come back to the starting position. This exercise is done quickly to let your core muscles generate some power.

6. Repeat the movement 10–15 times to complete one set. Do two to three sets, with about a minute of rest in between.

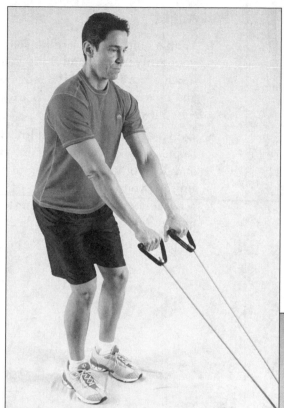

Starting/ending position.

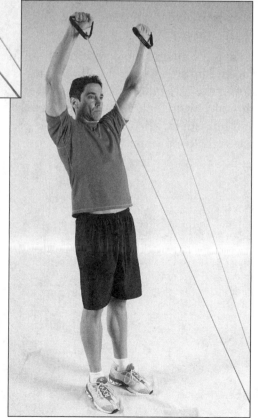

Midpoint position.

Forward Chop

Chopping wood is an excellent example of a chore that really requires the use of the core muscles. The forward chop exercise mimics the motion of cutting wood and gets all the same core muscles involved, without the need to build a fire when you're done. This exercise is the exact opposite of the stump puller, using the big latisimus dorsi (lats) muscles of the back to generate lots of power. You will again be using speed with this exercise, so prepare to get your heart rate up.

Preparation

1. Loop your resistance tubing through your door anchor or over a pole above your head. Hold one handle in each hand.

2. Facing the anchor, hold your hands up in the air and step back until all the slack is out of the tubing. Stand with your feet shoulder-width apart, with your knees and hips slightly bent. You should be prepared to "chop some wood."

Movement

3. With a quick downward movement, keep your arms straight and bring your hands down toward the floor. Bend your knees and hips so that your hands are about a foot above the floor.

4. Don't stop here. Quickly allow the tubing to pull you back to the starting position, and do another repetition until you have finished your set. Three sets of 10–15 reps will be plenty to get your heart rate going. Rest about a minute between sets.

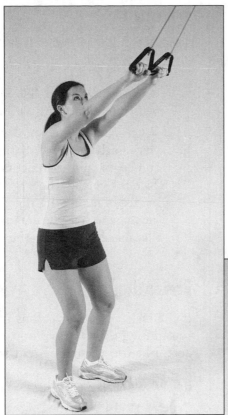

Starting/ending position.

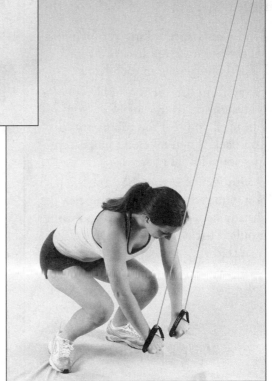

Midpoint position.

Overhead Pull

The overhead pull takes us back to a smaller movement that engages most of the core muscles as stabilizers. The resistance during the exercise will be really high because the tubing is going to be as far away from your core muscles as it can get. This exercise is a great assistance exercise that will enhance your ability to generate power and strength during stump pullers and forward chops, as well as some of the more advanced moves in later chapters. This is a foundation exercise that you will really feel working but that won't get you quite as tired as some of the others.

Preparation

1. Loop your resistance tubing through your door anchor or over a pole above your head. Hold one handle in each hand.

2. Face away from the anchor, hold your hands straight up over your head, and step out until you feel the tubing try to pull you back. Then take one more step to apply some initial resistance.

3. Stand with your feet together. In this position, your core abdominal muscles will already be working to keep you from being pulled backward, but the exercise hasn't started yet.

Movement

4. Keeping your hands above your head and your arms straight, slowly pull the tubing until you can just see it in front of you without looking up. The resistance will really be pulling you back at this point.

5. When you can see your hands in front of you, slowly let it back to the starting point and begin another repetition immediately. Notice that the whole movement is just a matter of inches. It's not the size of the movement, but the amount of resistance that makes this exercise excellent.

Precautions

If you feel any pain or pulling in your lower back during this exercise, stop and consult your doctor before attempting it again. Don't do this exercise quickly. It is meant to be done slowly so that the core muscles really work to stabilize your body.

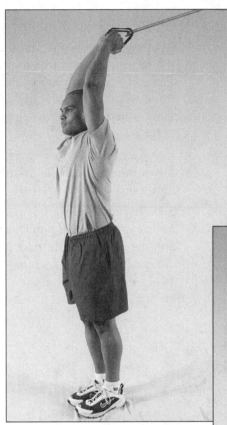

Starting/ending position.

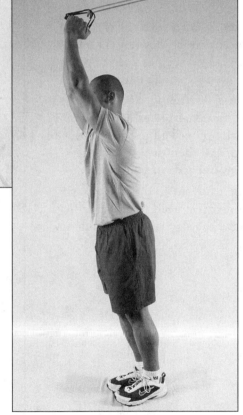

Midpoint position.

Kneeling Ground Throw

This exercise is a variation of the stump puller exercise. Instead of standing, you are kneeling. This effectively reduces your initial stability by taking any help your leg muscles may provide out of the equation, which makes the core muscles work even harder. On top of that, the motion also includes some rotation, so you'll get even more core-conditioning results out of this one.

Preparation

1. Attach your resistance tubing through your door anchor at foot level or under something heavy, such as a leg of your couch. Hold one handle in each hand.

2. Kneel facing the tubing. You may want to use an exercise mat to cushion your knees. Back up until all the slack is out of the tubing, and then turn so that the anchor is to one side of your body.

3. Hold both arms out to the side toward the anchor. If you need to move farther away to take the slack out of the tubing, do it now.

Movement

4. Keeping your arms straight, quickly pull the tubing up and across your body. Pretend you are trying to throw something from the ground into the air and away from you (such as when you're pulling weeds).

5. Let the tubing pull you back to the starting point, and perform another repetition until your set is complete.

6. Switch directions so that you are starting on the other side of your body, and do another set here. Alternate sides until you are done. Four sets (two on each side) of 10–15 reps will suffice.

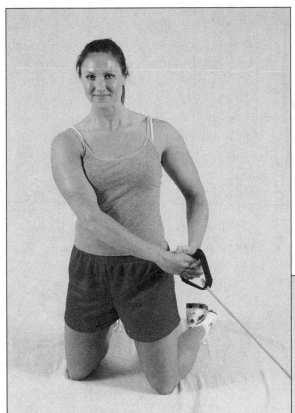

Starting/ending position.

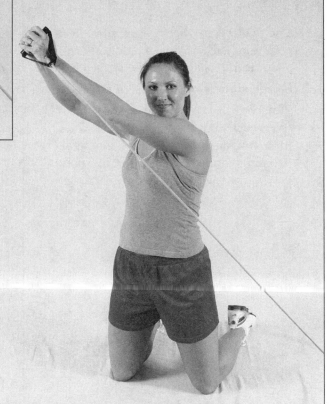

Midpoint position.

Kneeling Cross Chop

As with the kneeling ground throw, this exercise is harder than its cousin, the forward chop, because the assistance of the leg muscles has been removed and there is a new component of rotation. Your core abdominal muscles are really going to get a workout now, and they are being joined by the big back muscles and some shoulder stabilizers. The kneeling cross chop will get your blood flowing because you will be doing these rather quickly to build core power and strength. Move only as fast as you can while still maintaining control over the tubing.

Preparation

1. Loop your resistance tubing through your door anchor or over a pole above your head. Hold one handle in each hand.

2. Kneel on the floor in front of the tubing.

3. Hold your hands over your head, and scoot back until there isn't any slack left in the tubing. The resistance should be pulling you up and forward at this point.

Movement

4. Keeping your arms straight, quickly pull both hands down and across your body to the floor outside your left knee (don't slam your hands into the floor, though).

5. As soon as the tubing is down, let it back up and quickly pull it down and across your body to the floor outside your right knee.

6. Repeat chops to the left and right until you've done 5–10 reps on each side. Rest 15–20 seconds and repeat until four sets are complete.

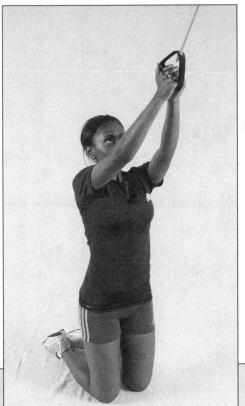

Starting/ending position.

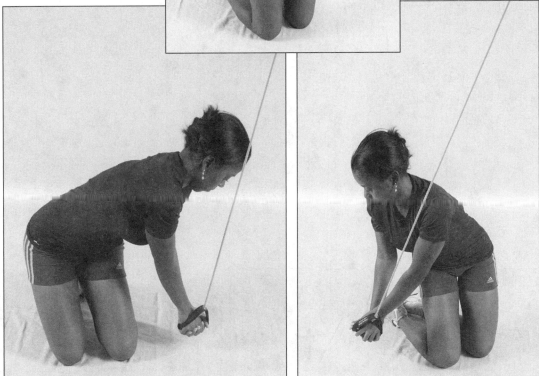

Left midpoint position.

Right midpoint position.

In This Chapter

- ◆ Adding balance to the resistance
- ◆ Throwing with tubing
- ◆ The Russian exercise
- ◆ Pulling with your legs

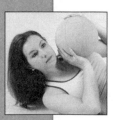
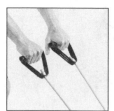
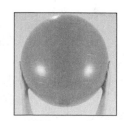
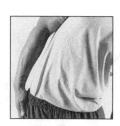
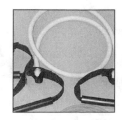
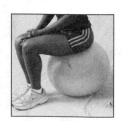

Advanced Resistance Tubing Exercises

Love it or hate it, you have to admit by now that resistance tubing really does make core conditioning that much better. The last chapter gave you a taste of what is possible, and it just keeps getting better. In this chapter, you will learn some of the more advanced resistance tubing exercises for the core. The component of balance is back in the mix, and there are more power movements. I'll bet you just can't wait (can't wait to be done with your workout, that is)!

I've finished my peanut butter and jelly sandwich, and now it's time to work off some of that—no rest for the weary. You are about to learn how to balance, stabilize, pull, push, and power your way through a great workout. Make sure you have mastered the exercises in Chapter 6 before you move into these advanced moves. The core is a tricky thing: great exercises will make it even better, but if you aren't ready, an injury is just one move away. Tackle this chapter with confidence if the last chapter has you feeling a little bored. I'll see you and your even stronger core on the other side.

Resisted Side Bend

Remember those side bends you did back in Chapter 4? Well, it's time to bring them back and make them more challenging. The original side bends worked the muscles of the abdominals and lower back against the force of gravity. Now we are going to use gravity plus resistance tubing to double the fun. This exercise is all about stability and movement. One side of your body will be pulling, and the other side will be getting pulled. Focus on keeping your body moving from side to side in smooth motions, and you'll quickly notice how your posture improves. With practice, resisted side bends will allow you to carry heavy objects in both hands without straining your shoulders.

Preparation

1. Stand with your feet shoulder-width apart.

2. Loop your resistance tubing under both feet and grab the handles on each side. There shouldn't be any slack in the tubing. If there is, spread your feet a little farther apart, or wrap the tubing around your hand once on each side.

Movement

3. Slowly lean over to one side, running your hand down the side of your leg as far as you can go without losing your balance. As one arm is going down, the other arm is pulling up on the tubing. Keep the pulling arm against the side of your body; don't try to pull it up by bending your elbow—just let your core do the work.

4. Return to the upright position and lean over to the other side as far as you can.

5. Keep your hand against the side of your body at all times. This will ensure that you are bending to the side, not forward or backward.

6. Complete 10–15 bends on each side for one set. Do three or four sets for a complete workout.

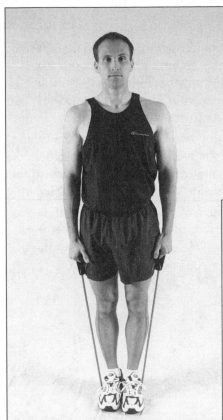

Starting/ending position.

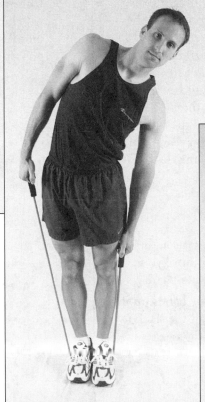

Left midpoint position.

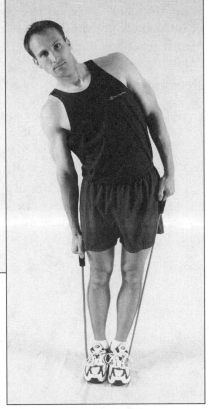

Right midpoint position.

Diagonal Wood Chop

Have you ever seen a lumberjack with a weak core? Probably not—those guys are usually very strong and sturdy. With the diagonal wood chop, you use a lot of power and rotation to enlist the work of a ton of your core muscles— and gain the strength of a lumberjack yourself. The big back muscles, shoulder stabilizers, hip flexors, and abdominals are all going to be working. This exercise is pretty strenuous, so make sure you have caught your breath from your last exercise before you begin. Keep the image in your mind that you are chopping wood, an activity that takes a lot of energy and power. You want to duplicate that activity and get your core moving and building strength. You will notice at the bottom of the movement that the intensity moves higher as the tubing is being stretched. This is where you really want to be in control and make those muscles do exactly what you want.

Preparation

1. Loop your resistance tubing through your door anchor or over a pole above your head. Hold one handle in each hand.

2. Facing the anchor, hold your hands up in the air and step back until all the slack is out of the tubing. Stand with your feet shoulder-width apart, with your knees and hips slightly bent.

Movement

3. With a quick downward movement, keep your arms straight and bring your hands down toward the floor outside your left foot. Bend your knees and hips so that you get down to about a foot above the floor.

4. Don't stop here. Quickly allow the tubing to pull you back to the starting position, and do another repetition down toward the floor outside your right foot and back up.

5. Continue alternating left and right diagonal chops until you have finished 10 reps on each side. That's one set, two more to go (after you rest a few seconds).

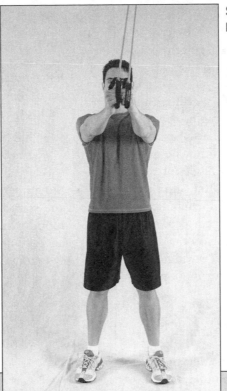

Starting/ending position.

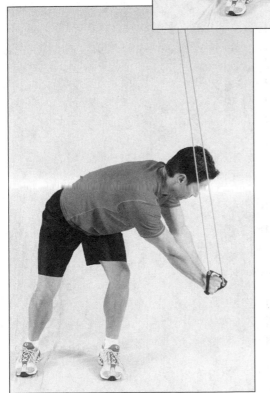

Left midpoint position.

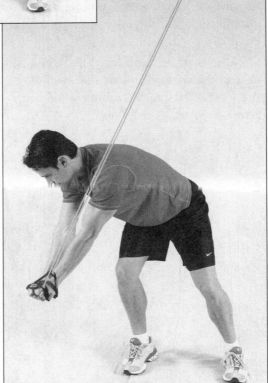

Right midpoint position.

Balanced Side Pull

Now you are going to use the resistance tubing to work on stabilization and rotation in a very slow and controlled exercise. The balanced side pull doesn't involve any power or speed. It's all about slowly and consistently engaging the core muscles to keep you balanced while the arms move through their range of motion. The exercise won't do much for the arm muscles; it isn't supposed to. It's the core we are after, and that's just what you are going to get. Maintaining balance while your core is moving against a resistance is one of the hardest things you can ask your body to do. With practice, you will feel very smooth and in control of your motions—that's core conditioning.

Preparation

1. Attach one end of your resistance tubing to your door anchor or around a pole at chest level. Hold the other end in the one hand.

2. Stand so that the hand with the tubing is next to the anchor, and step away until there is no slack in the tubing while your arm is held out to the side.

Movement

3. If the tubing is in your right hand, stand on your right foot. If the tubing is in your left hand, stand on your left foot. After a set on one side, you will switch and do a set on the other side.

4. Keeping your arm straight and at shoulder level, slowly pull the tubing until your arm is pointing straight out in front of you.

5. Slowly return the arm back to your side and start a new repetition. Don't put your foot down between reps—keep that balance. Finish 10–15 reps in one set before switching sides and doing another set. Complete a total of two sets on each side.

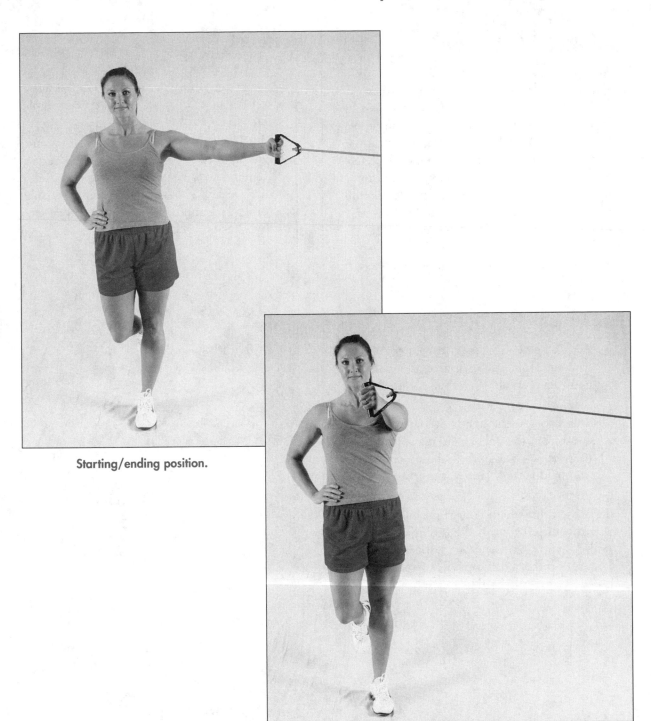

Starting/ending position.

Midpoint position.

Balanced Cross-Pull

Like the balanced side pull, this exercise is important for building stabilization and balance. All the same muscles are involved here, just in a new direction. Instead of pulling the tubing toward your body, you will be pulling it away from your body. This is an extra challenge because the tubing will be getting longer and longer, which means harder and harder. You'll also be balancing on the opposite leg from the arm you use to pull, so this makes your core work on both sides at the same time. I'm sure you're up to the challenge by now, so take it slowly and concentrate on standing still.

Preparation

1. Attach one end of your resistance tubing to your door anchor or around a pole at chest level. Hold the other end in the one hand.

2. Stand so that the hand with the tubing is away from the anchor. Step away until there is no slack in the tubing, with your arm held straight across the front of your body.

3. If the tubing is in your right hand, stand on your left foot. If the tubing is in your left hand, stand on your right foot. After a set on this side, you will switch and do a set on the other side.

Movement

4. Keeping your arm straight, slowly pull on the tubing until your arm is pointed out to your side. This is a full 180 degrees of movement for the arm.

5. Slowly return to the starting position and complete 10–15 repetitions for this set. Remember to keep that foot in the air— don't let it down. Switch to the other side (other arm and hand) and do another set. Two sets on each side is perfect.

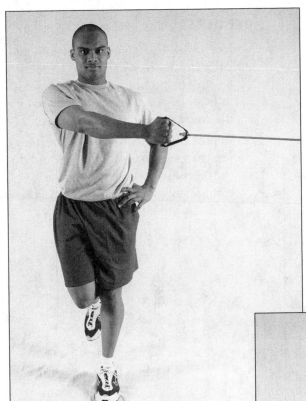

Starting/ending position.

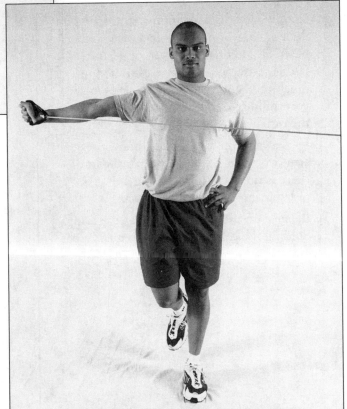

Midpoint position.

One-Arm Throw

The one-arm throw continues to build on your balancing skill. Now the resistance is going to be over your head instead of right next to you. Remember what happens when the resistance moves way up over your head? It stretches your body and makes your core muscles work even harder. This exercise also adds power and coordination. With the resistance on only one arm, you'll tend to be a bit off-balance as you learn this move. Concentrate on keeping your core and body still as only your arm moves. It will be a challenge, but this is what core conditioning is all about.

Preparation

1. Loop your resistance tubing through your door anchor or over a pole above your head. Hold both handles in one hand. If this resistance level proves to be too much to begin with, reattach one end of your tubing to the anchor and hold on to the other end of it.

2. Face away from the anchor, hold your arm over your head, and step away until there is no slack in the tubing and it is just starting to pull you backward.

3. Balance on the same-side leg as the arm holding the tubing (right arm equals right leg, left arm equals left leg).

Movement

4. Keep your body upright and still, and your arm perfectly straight. Quickly pull on the tubing until your arm is pointing in front of you, and quickly return it to the starting position.

5. Repeat these throws 10–15 times for one set; then switch arms and legs and do another set. Two sets on each arm/leg combo will give you the results you want.

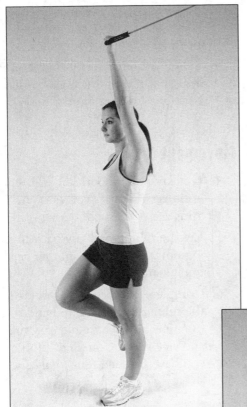

Starting/ending position.

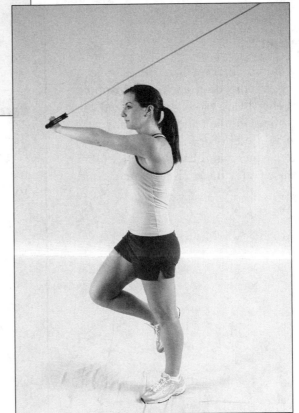

Midpoint position.

Two-Arm Throw

This exercise adds something you haven't experienced yet: different resistance for each side of your body. The two-arm throw is similar to the one-arm throw, in that it is difficult but very beneficial. At the same time, it's different because you will be using two different sizes of resistance tubing (one in each hand). Get ready to really feel your core working against the tubing and against itself. This is where the exercise gets interesting. One side of the body will be working against a harder resistance tube, but the easy side has to pick up the pace to stabilize the core because it's going to want to rotate. This sounds a bit confusing, so let's just get to it so you can feel what I'm talking about.

Preparation

1. Attach two different sizes of resistance tubing to your door anchor or to a pole over your head. Hold the other end of the tubing in one hand. Each hand will have a different tube in it, and it doesn't matter which hand has the harder tubing, because you will switch for your second set.

2. Face away from the anchor, hold your hands over your head, and step away until the slack is out of both tubes.

3. Stand with your feet a couple of inches apart but right next to each other (don't have one foot behind the other).

Movement

4. Quickly pull on both tubes, keeping your arms as straight as you can, until both arms are pointing directly in front of you.

5. Let the tubing pull you back to the starting point, and begin another repetition immediately.

6. Complete 10–15 reps in a set; then switch the tubing from hand to hand so the hard tubing is now where the easy tubing was, and vice versa. Complete another set until you have finished four total sets.

Variations

To make this exercise even harder, balance on one foot—it doesn't matter which. This will really work your core and get more of your hip rotator muscles involved in the stabilization.

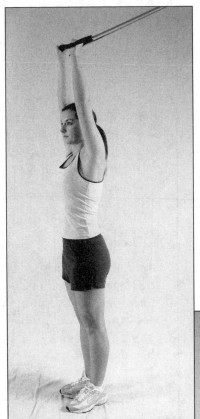

Starting/ending position.

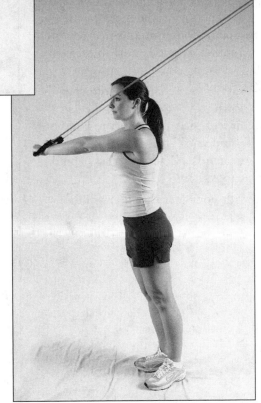

Midpoint position.

Granny Pass

No, this exercise doesn't involve your grandmother—unless you are teaching her how to do it. The granny pass is named after the old "granny"-style basketball shot, an underhand shot you never see anymore. This is really a mirror image of the two-arm throw, except that you will be using only one resistance tube. Because you will be pulling from the bottom instead of from the top, the lower-back muscles will get into this a whole lot more. As you've seen before, stabilization will be a key component here. You've just got to stand still and move at the same time. Sounds easy, right?

Preparation

1. Loop your resistance tubing through your door anchor or under the leg of your couch or something heavy at ground level. Hold on to one handle in each hand.

2. Face away from the anchor, hold your hands down to your sides, and step away until you feel the tubing start to pull your arms behind you. Take one more step so that your hands are actually just behind your buttocks.

3. Stand with your feet shoulder-width apart.

Movement

4. Keeping your arms straight, quickly pull with both hands until your arms are pointing out in front of you and just above parallel to the floor.

5. Let the tubing pull you back to the starting position, and begin another repetition immediately. Finish 10–15 reps per set for three sets, resting 15–20 seconds between each set.

Variations

You can make this exercise even more challenging if you stand on one foot. Having to balance during an exercise always makes the core muscles work harder. Alternate your standing leg for each set so one side doesn't get more work than the other.

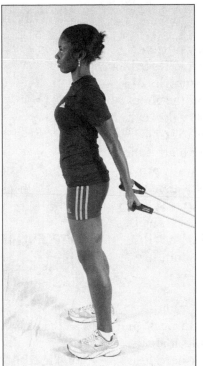

Starting/ending position.

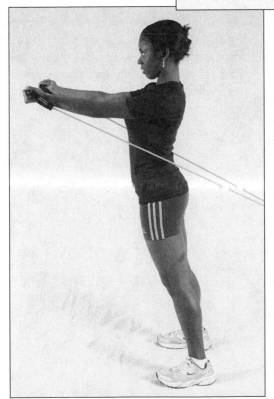

Midpoint position.

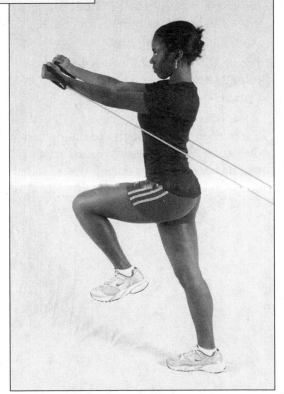

Variation standing on one foot.

Lying Leg Pull

Now it's time for something really different: using the resistance tubing with your legs. This exercise goes after the large core muscles of the hip extensors, mostly found in the glutes. Additionally, the abdominals and back extensor muscles will be working together to stabilize your upper body while your lower body is moving. The resistance tubing won't really provide a lot of challenge for your legs—that's not the idea. It's your core we are going after, so that's where the work will be done. You will feel this exercise more in the abs and lower back than the hips—that's exactly what you want.

Preparation

1. Loop your resistance tubing through your door anchor or around a pole at about shoulder height. If you are using a heavy resistance tube, it may be better to use a pair of lighter ones because the tubing really gets stretched during this exercise.

2. Lie on the floor, facing away from the tubing anchor. Keep your arms down at your sides.

3. Raise your legs into the air, and slide the toe of each foot through the tubing handles as far as possible. To make sure the handles don't slip off during the exercise, keep your toes pointed.

Movement

4. In a slow, controlled movement, pull down with both feet until they just touch the floor.

5. Slowly return to the starting position and begin another repetition immediately. Really focus on your slow movement; this is not about power, but control and stabilization. Do three sets of 10–15 repetitions, resting 15–20 seconds between sets.

Precautions

If you feel any pain or "pulling" in your lower back during this exercise, stop and consult with your doctor. You may not be ready for this one yet.

Variations

You can perform this exercise one leg at a time. Just keep one foot in the air while you pull down with the other leg. Alternating left and right legs creates some rotation you will have to stabilize against, but that just means you will get more results!

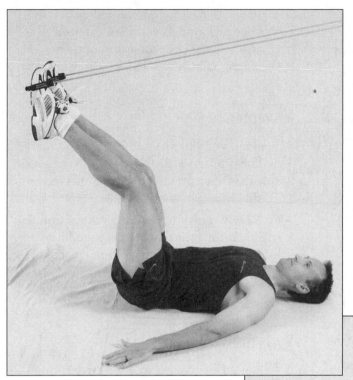

Starting/ending position.

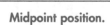

Midpoint position.

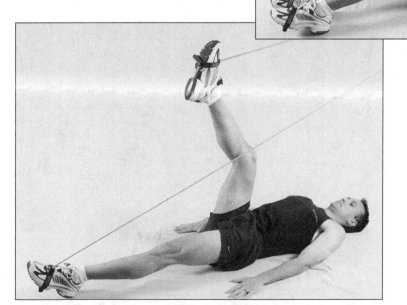

Variation with alternating legs.

Lying Tuck

The lying tucks work the hip flexors instead of the hip extensors—exactly the opposite of the lying leg pulls (see how we keep creating a balanced workout?). This exercise also focuses on stabilizing the torso while the legs are moving and the hip flexors are working their guts out. Stay in control of the movement and tubing at all times during this exercise—don't get caught up in wanting to do more reps than you can by sacrificing form to get there. You'll feel this one in your abdominals and in your hips. Although your thighs and hamstrings may get tired, too, they aren't the focus of this exercise.

Preparation

1. Loop your resistance tubing through your door anchor or under the leg of your couch or something heavy at floor level.

2. Sit on the floor facing the anchor. Slide the tubing handles over your feet as far as you can. Keep your feet pointed toward the ceiling so the tubing doesn't slide off.

3. Scoot back until all the slack is out of the tubing.

4. Prop yourself up on your elbows. Use your abdominals and back extensor muscles to keep your torso straight—no sagging allowed!

Movement

5. Bend your knees and hips to pull your knees up toward your chest as far as you can. Don't try to yank them up—move slowly and in control.

6. Slowly return to the starting position, but don't put your feet back on the floor. Start another repetition immediately. Do 10–15 repetitions per set for three sets. Rest 15–20 seconds between each set.

Variations

To make this exercise a wee bit harder, alternate the legs right and left instead of together, and don't let them rest on the floor between reps. This variation will make one side work while the other side stabilizes the movement.

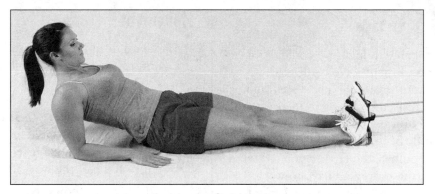

Starting/ending position.

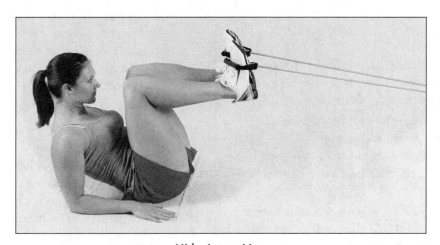

Midpoint position.

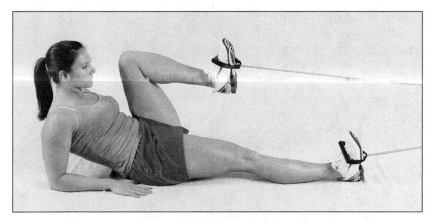

Variation with alternating legs.

Resisted Sit-Up

By now you probably thought we couldn't make sit-ups any more difficult. Well, guess what? We're only getting started! The resisted sit-ups shown here use resistance tubing to increase the difficulty of the upward portion of the movement, and that difficulty increases the farther up you sit. Remember, the farther you stretch a resistance tube, the more you have to work. In this case, as you sit up, it will get harder and harder the higher you get. Cool, huh?

Preparation

1. Loop your resistance tubing through your door anchor or under the leg of something heavy at floor level.

2. Lie on an exercise mat or carpeted surface, with your head closest to the tubing anchor. Bend your knees so that your feet are no more than a foot away from your butt.

3. Grab hold of the tubing, with one handle in each hand. Hold the handles next to your shoulders, keeping your elbows at your sides.

4. Scoot away from the anchor until all the slack is out of the tubing. Anchor your feet under something heavy, or have a friend hold them.

Movement

5. Take a deep breath in, and as you blow it out, roll your head and shoulders off the ground toward your knees (this is basically an abdominal crunch so far). When your shoulders leave the floor, keep your abdominals contracted and begin pulling with the hip flexor muscles to bring your entire back all the way off the floor.

6. Touch your elbows to your knees, and slowly lower yourself back to the floor.

7. When you can do three sets of 30 reps, your core will be in excellent shape. If you can't do 30 reps right away, just do as many as you can each set, and rest about a minute between sets.

Variations

Of course, you can make this harder: don't anchor your feet. If you aren't ready for that yet, you can combine this with the modified sit-up (see Chapter 5) by holding one leg in the air while the other leg is anchored down.

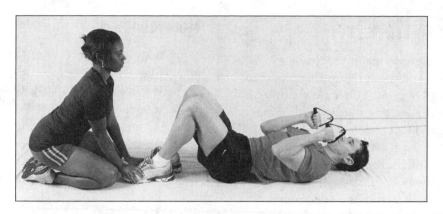

Starting/ending position.

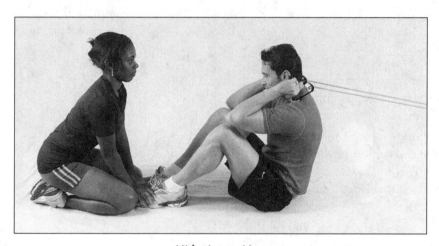

Midpoint position.

Seated Russian Twist

Whether this exercise was invented by a Russian, I don't know, but that's what it's called, so let's just work with it. What I do know is that this very challenging core-conditioning exercise is all about rotation. Getting back to creating power, the Russian twist uses the abdominal core muscles for movement and the back extensors for stabilization. The back has to work continually, while the abdominals alternate from side to side. You can really get your heart rate up doing these, but always stay in control of your speed.

Preparation

1. Loop your resistance tubing through your door anchor or around a pole at ground level.

2. Sit on the floor facing the anchor. Hold one end of the tubing in each hand, and hug your arms to your chest. Scoot away from the anchor until all the slack is out of the tubing.

3. Keep your legs straight and your feet pointed toward the ceiling. Sit up as straight as you can during the entire exercise.

Movement

4. Moving to either side, start slowly and rotate your torso as far as you can. Then return to the starting point and continue rotating to the other side as far as you can.

5. As you get the hang of this exercise, increase the speed of your rotations to make it more difficult. Always keep your torso straight and your arms to your chest.

6. Alternate left and right rotations until you have completed a set of 10 reps to each side. Complete three sets, resting 15–20 seconds before starting the next set.

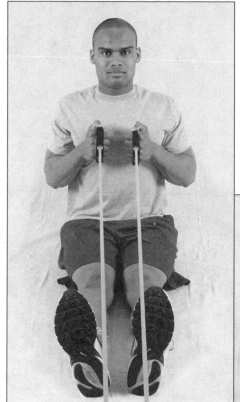

Starting/ending position.

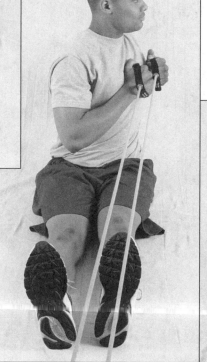

Left midpoint position.

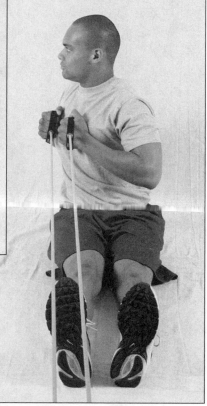

Right midpoint position.

In This Chapter

◆ Gaining momentum

◆ Toss a ball around

◆ Exercises with power and bounce

◆ Another level of crunch

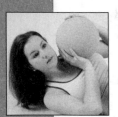
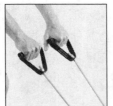
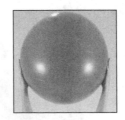
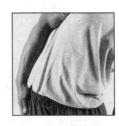
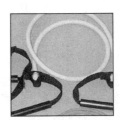
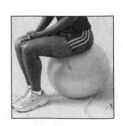

Chapter 8

Beginning Medicine Ball Exercises

Take two of these and exercise in the morning! I'm not talking about aspirin, but one of the oldest exercise tools ever prescribed: medicine balls. Why are they called medicine balls? Beats me. I spent quite a bit of time researching this and even had a couple of students work on it for extra credit, all to no avail. What I do know is that, no matter what you call them—medicine balls, heavy balls, or resistance balls—they work. The secret (don't tell anyone I told you) to medicine balls is that they add the force of momentum to your core-conditioning program. Momentum is a force that you have to work against to make it stop moving. The faster you move a medicine ball, the harder you have to work to make it stop moving. Your core muscles have to produce the force to get it moving and then to make it stop—so it's almost twice the exercise!

Don't blame me for making it harder—blame physics. A basic law of physics states that "an object in motion will stay in motion." You gotta love science; it gives us all kinds of new ways to make your core muscles stronger than ever. As you work through this chapter, you will come to understand how your core can work in more than one way at a time. You will feel a lot of muscles working that you didn't think you could work. You may have not even known you could feel them until now. You'll also get a chance to do something you probably haven't done since you were a kid: play with balls.

Wood Chop

This exercise is a variation of the forward chop exercise you did with resistance tubing in Chapter 6. The wood chop is more like actually chopping wood because the medicine ball provides a resistance that's a whole lot like an axe: it wants to keep moving once you start swinging it. The wood chop introduces you to the effect momentum has on the muscles you use and how your core responds to this use. When you get the feel of this exercise, really go for speed and get those muscles contracting, stretching, and contracting again, and again, and again.

Preparation

1. Hold a medicine ball with both hands. Choose the size and weight of ball that is appropriate for your level of training and the intensity you want to achieve.

2. Stand with your feet slightly wider than shoulder-width apart. Make sure that one foot is not behind the other; they should be even (like you're standing on a line).

3. Hold the ball over your head, with your arms straight.

Movement

4. With as much speed as you can handle, quickly swing the ball down and through your legs. As you come down, bend your knees and hips to bring the ball down until it almost touches the ground as it swings through your legs.

5. Slow the ball down and quickly reverse your motion, swinging the ball back up in the air over your head. During this entire motion, your arms should stay straight.

6. Repeat swinging down and up until you have finished 10–15 repetitions for one set. Rest 15–20 seconds before your next set.

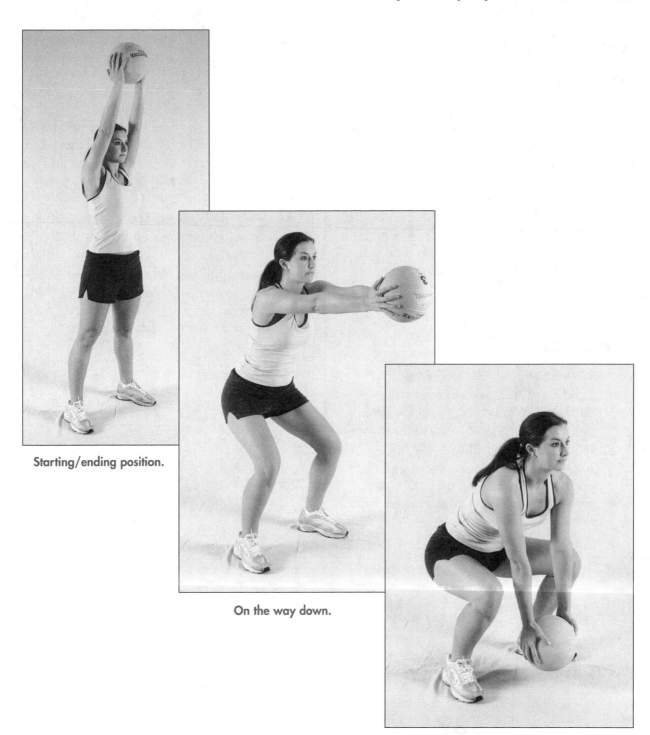

Starting/ending position.

On the way down.

Midpoint position.

Crunch Twist

This exercise combines two easier exercises and adds the resistance of a medicine ball to really bring your abdominals to life. The crunch twist is half crunch, half oblique crunch, and all fun. When you do this exercise while holding a medicine ball under your chin, you are effectively increasing the weight your abdominals have to lift off the floor. When you twist to the side to get the obliques firing, the medicine ball adds to the rotating mass that has to be accelerated and decelerated. Basically, this means that your core abdominal muscles are going to be pushed to work harder than ever, giving you an even stronger core.

Preparation

1. Lie on your back on the floor.
2. Bend your knees and slide your feet up until they are no more than a foot from your butt. Keep your feet flat on the floor.
3. Hold a medicine ball with the appropriate weight and size for your ability right under your chin. Hold the ball in place with both hands, and always keep it firmly pressed against your chest.

Movement

4. Take a deep breath in. As you blow it out, roll your head and shoulders up off the floor into a crunched position.
5. When your shoulder blades are fully off the floor, hold your abdominals tight, and rotate as far to one side as you can and then back to the middle. Speed up your rotation as you master this movement.
6. Slowly lower yourself back to the floor. Take another breath, and repeat the crunch and twist to the other side.
7. Repeat until you have done 15 crunch twists to each side, resting for about 2 seconds (one deep breath) between each crunch. Do two or three sets.

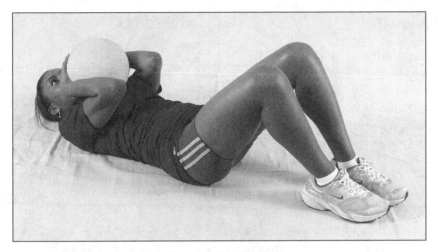

Starting/ending position.

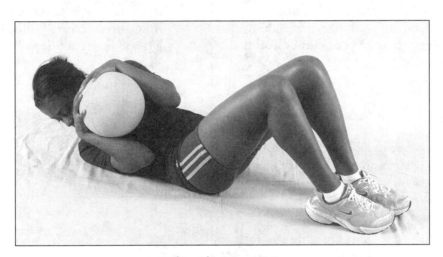

Right midpoint position.

Stump Throw

Stump throws are a combination of a stump puller (see Chapter 6) and a wood chop done in reverse, with the addition of a twist at the end just for good measure. When you are cleaning out the garage and it's time to give something the old heave-ho, this exercise will come in handy. This exercise involves a lot of muscles as you bend down, stand up, and swing a medicine ball up and over one shoulder. The glutes, back, and shoulders are the main muscles working in the core, with the obliques and abdominals assisting the rotation and deceleration of the trunk. You'll really feel a good stretch at the midpoint of this exercise and, immediately after that, a strong contraction of the abdominals. Nearly everything in your core is working during this exercise, so results should come quickly.

Preparation

1. Hold a medicine ball with both hands. Choose the size and weight of ball that is appropriate for your level of training and the intensity you want to achieve.

2. Stand with your feet slightly shoulder-width apart. Make sure that one foot is not behind the other; they should be even (like you're standing on a line).

3. Hold the ball down in front of you, arms straight. Squat down until the ball just touches the floor.

Movement

4. Quickly stand up and, at the same time, swing the ball up and out in an arc in front of you. As the ball is coming up, angle it to one side a bit so that at the top of the swing, when the ball is all the way above you, it is traveling over one shoulder (either left or right—it doesn't matter).

5. At the top of the swing, slow the ball down as it passes over your shoulder, and pull it back down in the same arc, keeping your arms straight.

6. Bring the ball all the way back to the starting point, letting your hips and knees bend to get back to the squatting position. Immediately change directions and begin another repetition, but to the other shoulder.

7. Repeat stump throws over the left and right shoulders until you have completed 20 total repetitions. Rest 15–20 seconds before your next set.

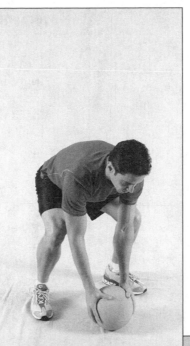

Starting/ending position.

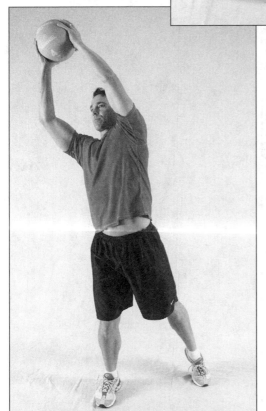

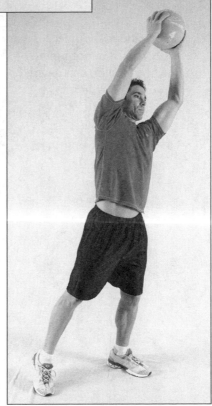

Right side midpoint position.

Left side midpoint position.

Slam Dunk

By now you've probably found that the medicine ball really does add a new level of resistance to your core-conditioning program. Now you get to have a little bit of revenge against the ball. In the slam dunk exercise, you won't be using a basketball, and you don't have to jump very high—actually, not at all. This exercise is all about creating a lot of power, moving quickly, and reacting to the momentum the ball creates. Make sure you have quite a bit of open space around you for this exercise. If the ball gets away from you, it is probably going to go on a destructive rampage. You may even want to go out to the garage or driveway, where you can do this on pavement or somewhere with a high ceiling, in case you miss the catch.

Preparation

1. Stand with your feet about shoulder-width apart. Hold the ball in both hands over your head as high as you can reach. Keep a firm grasp on both sides of the ball because you are getting ready to throw it to the ground.

Movement

2. With lots of speed and power, quickly throw the ball down toward the ground right in front of you. Release the ball once it gets to about waist level—don't bend down toward the ground.

3. The ball should hit the ground right in front of you and bounce straight back up. As it is coming back up, catch it and let the momentum of the ball carry you back to the starting position.

4. When you get the ball back over your head, slam it down again. Repeat slam dunks until you have completed 10–15 repetitions. Rest for a few seconds and do two more sets.

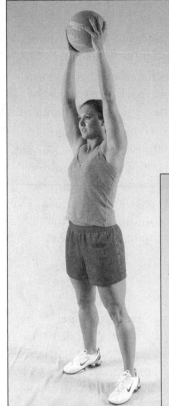

Starting/ending position.

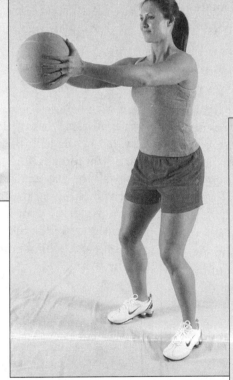

Release/catch position.

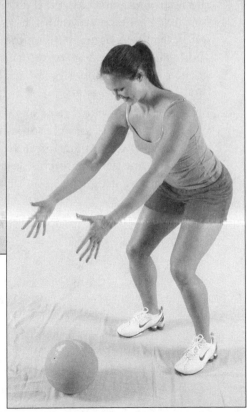

Midpoint position—ball hits the floor.

Russian Twist

You've seen the Russian twist done with resistance tubing, but this is the original exercise that started the craze. The Russian twist is all about rotation, so the core abdominals and lower-back muscles do the majority of the work. The medicine ball adds momentum to the twist, making the muscles work to accelerate you in one direction, and then work to slow you down at the end of the rotation and bring you back the other way. You will really feel the core muscles stretch at the end of each rotation and then contract in a flash to get you moving the other way quickly.

Preparation

1. Stand with your feet slightly wider than shoulder-width apart. Bend the knees and hips just a little bit so you are not standing perfectly straight. Bending the knees and hips allows the legs to absorb some of the rotation, keeping your back from doing too much twisting.

2. Hold the appropriate size of medicine ball for your ability and the intensity you want to generate straight out in front of you. Keep one hand on each side of the ball, squeezing it tight.

Movement

3. Keep your feet in place. Quickly rotate your body to the left as far as you can.

4. When you get as much twist as you can out of your trunk, quickly rotate all the way around to the right as far as you can.

5. Repeat rotations to the left and right as fast as you can with proper form. Keep the ball out in front of you at shoulder height. If the ball starts to sag, stop the exercise and rest, or use a lighter ball. Do 15–20 repetitions in each of three sets, resting about a minute between sets.

Precautions

The idea behind Russian twists is to get your core muscles working against the momentum created by the ball. Be careful not to let the ball carry you too far. The goal is not to twist your body all the way around, but just as far as you can while keeping the ball at shoulder height and not moving your legs any more than necessary. A good range of rotation is where the ball ends up just behind your shoulders at the end of the twist.

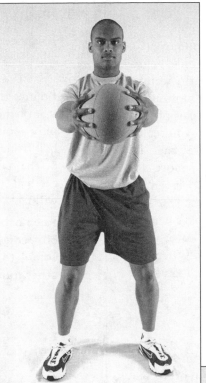

Starting/ending position.

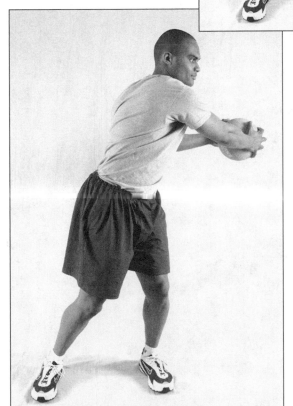

Left midpoint position.

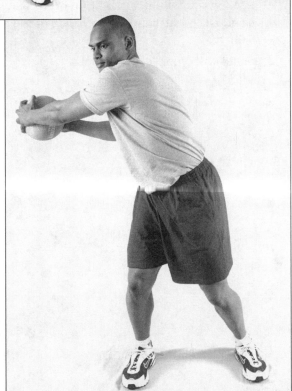

Right midpoint position.

Overhead Balance

This exercise doesn't involve a lot of movement, but it does involve a lot of muscle activation. During the overhead balance, the weight of the medicine ball, and the slight motion it will have, is going to make the muscles of your core react over and over again until you really start to feel the abdominals and lower back working as one unit. This exercise is more about stabilization than movement. Remember how the body works harder when the resistance is far away from the core? That's what you are doing here. Putting the ball over your head and standing on one foot makes the core muscles have to work constantly, giving you very impressive results.

Preparation

1. Hold a medicine ball of the appropriate size for your ability straight up over your head. Keep one hand on each side of the ball.

2. Stand with your feet together.

Movement

3. Balance on one foot. It doesn't matter which—you'll switch sides after the first set.

4. Bounce the medicine ball back and forth from hand to hand, keeping your hands only about a foot apart. Don't throw the ball from side to side; your hands won't be that far apart. The faster you bounce the ball from side to side, the more you will feel your core muscles working.

5. Keep balancing and bouncing for up to 60 seconds. Rest 15–20 seconds; then complete a set while balancing on the other foot. Finish two sets on each foot.

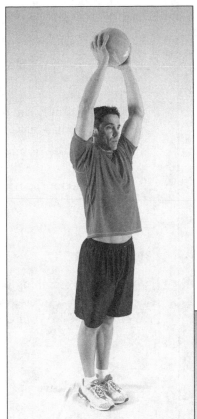

Starting/ending position.

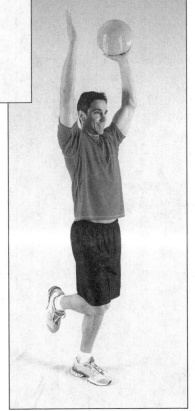

Midpoint position.

Prone Back Extension

The prone back extension is another stabilization exercise that doesn't involve a lot of movement but that will really push you to contract and hold your back muscles in place. This exercise targets the lower-back and deep posterior muscles, the upper back and shoulders, and a little bit of the glutes. This is one of the few exercises in which the core abdominals are not used; they get to rest (but don't start thinking this is going to be easy). This movement takes some practice to get good at. A lot of times, this exercise is used as a measure of lower-back strength in chiropractic and work-conditioning clinics. It is a very small movement, but with the resistance so far away from the body—well, you know how that works now.

Preparation

1. Lie face down on an exercise mat or carpeted surface.
2. Stretch your arms over your head. Hold a medicine ball of the appropriate size and weight for your ability in both hands, squeezing it from both sides. You probably won't need a very heavy ball to begin with, so start light and increase the weight as you master this exercise.

Movement

3. Lift the ball off the ground using your arms and shoulders. Lift your chest off the floor as high as you can. At the extreme range of this exercise, you will be able to lift only the top part of your chest off the floor—that's perfect.
4. Hold this position for up to 60 seconds. Relax back to the floor and rest for 15–20 seconds before starting the next set. Complete three to four sets.

Precautions

If you feel any cramping or pain in your lower back during this exercise, stop and relax. If the pain continues, see your doctor before you attempt it again.

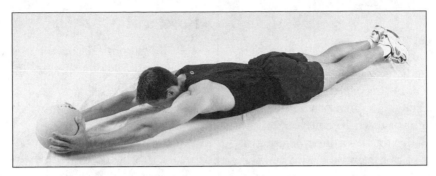

Starting/ending position.

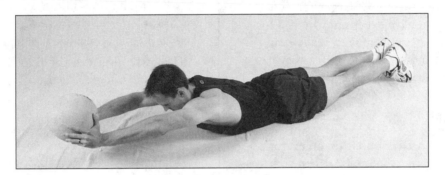

Midpoint position.

V-Sit

The V-sit is a combination of a sit-up and a pike, with the medicine ball providing a new level of resistance. In this exercise, you can do a sit-up without having to anchor your feet because the weight of the medicine ball will do that for you. Balance and coordination are going to be part of this exercise, so we will see how well you are progressing in those areas. During a V-sit, your core abdominals and hip flexors will work through a larger range of motion than you have experienced yet. This gives these muscles a chance to really strut their stuff and show you how much they can add to your solid core.

Preparation

1. Lie on your back on either an exercise mat or a carpeted surface. Keep your legs straight out and on the floor.

2. Place your medicine ball between your knees. Hold it there by squeezing it with both legs.

3. Cross your arms over your chest, with your fingertips touching your shoulders.

Movement

4. Keep your feet on the floor, and perform two thirds of a sit-up. Pull with your abdominals and hip flexors until your lower back is off the floor, but don't go all the way up.

5. When your upper body is about two thirds of the way up, lift your legs off the floor as high as you can while keeping them straight. You will probably lean back a little bit to maintain your balance; no problem there—just keep lifting your legs and your upper body as high as you can.

6. Slowly return to the floor and rest for a couple of deep breaths.

7. Repeat this move for 10–15 repetitions per set for three sets.

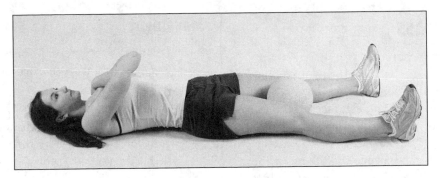

Starting/ending position.

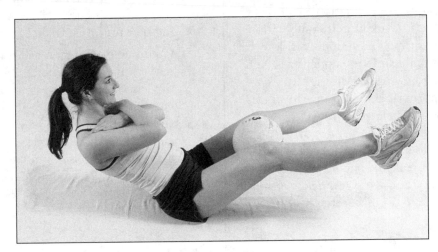

Midpoint position.

Balance Pass

For the next two exercises, you will need a partner to catch the ball and throw it back to you. If you can find someone who wants to do the exercise with you, you can face each other and toss the ball back and forth so each of you gets a workout. The balance pass is a measure of how well you can balance on one leg while your upper body reacts to catching, stopping, and throwing a medicine ball. Because the ball will be moving in a lot of directions, your core muscles will have to work in new combinations and at new intensities. The abdominals, lower back, hip flexor and extensors, upper back, and shoulders will all be working during this exercise. Find an appropriate space to perform this exercise. As you get stronger, you will need more space between you and your partner to throw the ball. It's a good idea to make sure there is nothing breakable behind you, in case you miss a catch. Your living room is probably not the best place to do this exercise.

Preparation

1. Stand with your feet together. Your partner should stand a couple feet from you. Your partner has the ball to start off.

Movement

2. Balance on one foot. When you feel balanced, signal to your partner to throw the ball to you.

3. Your partner should toss you the ball, either directly to your chest or just out to your left or right. The throw should not be hard—your partner should just get the ball to you.

4. Catch the ball in both hands. Stop it and then throw it back, all the while maintaining that precious balance.

5. Continue catching and throwing the ball until you have completed 10–15 repetitions in one set. Have your partner switch between throwing the ball to your chest and throwing it to the side. If you don't know which direction the ball is going, that makes this exercise even more fun and challenging. Rest for 15–20 seconds and balance on the other foot for the next set.

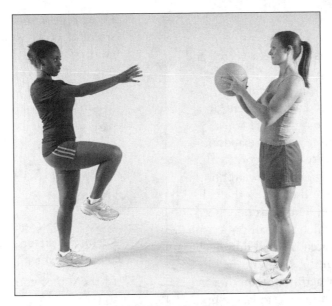

Starting/ending position.

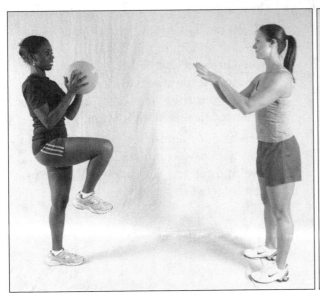

Catch at the chest.

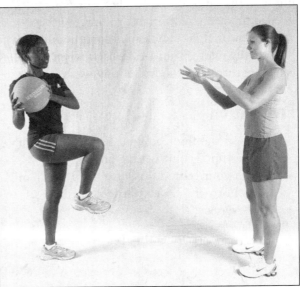

Catch to the side.

Sit-Up Throw

This exercise also requires a partner to catch and throw you the ball. Sit-up throws are another power exercise that uses the medicine ball to increase resistance and add a component of momentum for your core muscles to work with. During this exercise, your core abdominals are doing the majority of the work both as you come up and as you go down. Even though your arms are throwing and catching the ball, this isn't an arm exercise. The arms only get you into a position in which the ball can create resistance. When you catch the ball during the downward movement of the sit-up throw, the core muscles must contract more than they would if you were just doing a regular sit-up because the momentum and weight of the ball increase the amount of muscle involvement needed to keep you from just rolling over backward. I know this sounds a bit complicated, but it's actually a lot of fun—especially when you can start throwing the ball a long way.

Preparation

1. Lie on the floor on your back. Bend your knees until your feet are about 2 feet from your butt. This is farther away than you normally have your feet during a sit-up exercise.

2. Hold a medicine ball of the appropriate size and weight for your ability against your chest, just under your chin. Keep one hand on each side of the ball.

3. Your partner should stand a few feet away from your feet. The farther away your partner is, the more challenging this exercise becomes.

Movement

4. Keep the ball squeezed against your chest. Perform a sit-up using your abdominal and hip flexor muscles.

5. At the top of your sit-up, throw the ball to your partner.

6. Your partner will catch the ball and throw it right back to you, aiming for your chest.

7. Catch the ball out in front of you, absorb the momentum of the ball as you bring it to your chest, and lie back in the starting position. With practice, absorbing the ball to your chest as you go back down will become a smooth motion.

8. Repeat this exercise for 10–15 repetitions until you have completed your set. Do two to three sets with about a minute of rest in between.

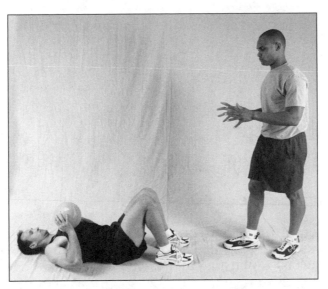

Starting/ending position.

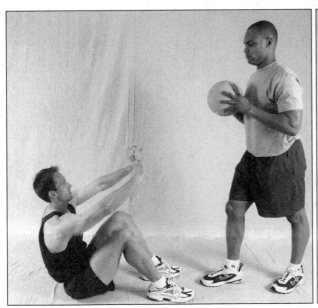

Midpoint position.

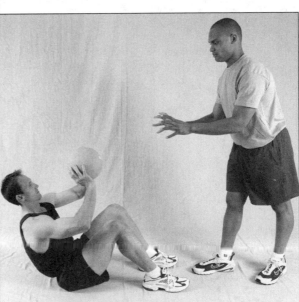

Catching the ball.

In This Chapter

- ◆ Throwing with power
- ◆ Training like a boxer
- ◆ Weighting down your rotations
- ◆ Exercising with a partner

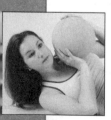
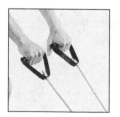
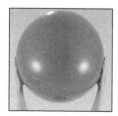
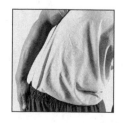
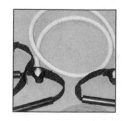
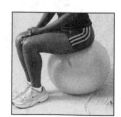

Chapter 9

Advanced Medicine Ball Exercises

Congratulations, you're halfway through the core-conditioning exercises. By now you've really learned a lot and are getting a good idea of where your core muscles are and how they work. Your workouts are starting to get more demanding, and you like it! As always, there is more to learn and do. This chapter takes medicine ball work one step further. The exercises you are about to see will push your core muscles to react and strengthen more. There really is no end to what they can do. The core muscles will take whatever you can throw at them.

Speaking of which, this chapter has a few more throwing exercises, so you can get a buddy involved in core conditioning. This is a great way to introduce core conditioning to your friends (other than buying them a copy of this book). They start out as your throwing partner, and pretty soon they want to be on the receiving end. Next thing you know, they're hooked. Now you can train together—pretty neat how that all works out.

Move through the exercises in this chapter after you have worked through Chapter 8. These exercises are a step above the beginning exercises and involve a lot more rotation, speed, and power development. As you gain strength and confidence in these workouts, increase the weight of your medicine ball to keep the improvements coming. You can buy medicine balls that weigh up to 50 pounds—although I don't recommend going that heavy unless you are entering a strongman competition or training for the Olympics. Keep the weight under 30 pounds, and your body will get the workout that it needs and wants.

Two-Hand Reach

The two-hand reach is a combination of stability and movement that focuses on a special action that gets your abdominal muscles working as hard as they can in a very short motion. I'd like to introduce your core muscles to the benefits of an eccentric action—that's basically a muscle "contraction" that occurs while the muscle is being stretched. Stretching and contracting at the same time is what makes you sore after a workout. You've done some of this in previous exercises, but just a little bit, so take it easy on this exercise at first.

Preparation

1. Stand with your feet together, heels and toes touching.
2. Hold your medicine ball in both hands, arms straight up over your head.

Movement

3. Keep your body stretched out as far as you can, and with a quick motion, press your hips forward and reach backward with your hands. This puts your body into a long arch that you will feel in your lower back as those muscles contract to move you.

4. As you move your hips forward and your arms back, your abdominal muscles will stretch. If you do the motion fast enough, you will automatically "bounce" back to the starting position. Help this motion along by contracting the abdominal muscles as much as you can.

5. Take a breath between each repetition. Do 10–15 repetitions as quickly as you can under control. Rest for a few moments and complete two to three total sets.

Precautions

If you feel any cramping or spasms in your lower back, discontinue this exercise until you have consulted with your doctor.

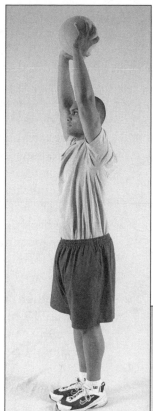

Starting/ending
position.

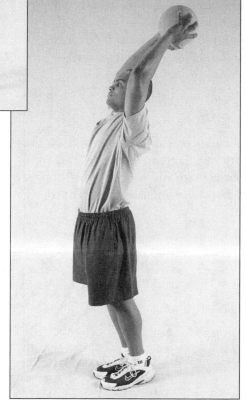

Midpoint position.

Walking Russian Twist

The walking Russian twist forces your core muscles into a position that they probably haven't been in before: really twisted up. The amount of rotation in this exercise is more than you have experienced so far. In this case, the hips will rotate one direction while the shoulders rotate another, effectively tying you in a big knot (just kidding). If you can imagine wringing out a wet towel, but the towel is actually your torso, with both ends being twisted in opposite directions, that's what you have here. Be aware of how your back feels during this exercise. Of all the exercises you have learned so far, this one poses the most risk of pushing you too far. Work within the limits of what you are able to do comfortably, and the results will creep up on you before you know it. You will need enough room to walk forward for at least 30 to 40 feet, so find a long hallway or walkway, or do this one outside.

Preparation

1. Hold a medicine ball straight out in front of you, with one hand on each side. Use the appropriate size and weight of ball for your ability and the intensity you want to create.

Movement

2. Take a giant step forward with one foot, like you are stepping over a large puddle of water.

3. With one foot out in front of you, rotate your body in the opposite direction your hips are facing. If your left foot is in front, rotate to your left. If your right foot is in front, rotate to your right. Make your rotation quick and powerful, moving as far as you can in that direction and quickly moving back to the front. The rotations should happen fast, almost as if you were going to throw the ball. Keep it straight out in front of you as much as you can.

4. Take another step and rotate in the other direction. Keep stepping until you have run out of room or done 30 steps, whichever comes first. Repeat two more times.

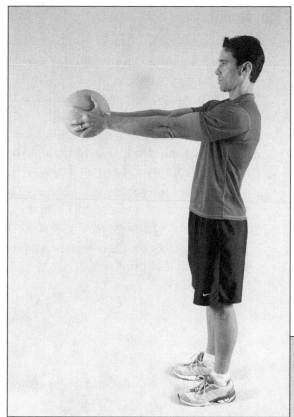

Starting/ending position.

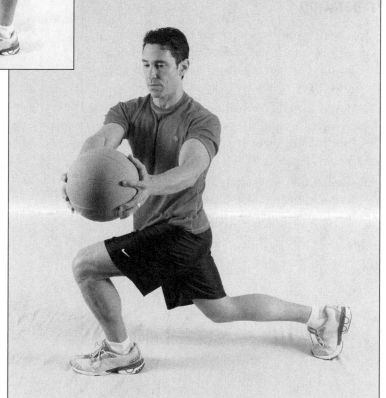

Left side midpoint position.

Lying Russian Twist

Just when you thought I couldn't come up with another way to combine the medicine ball and the Russian twist, here is the lying Russian twist (the next step is the upside-down combination twist with a twist while twisting—well, at least it sounds cool). This exercise adds even more resistance than holding the ball out in front of you. When you are standing, the weight of your upper body is balanced and supported by your legs. Now you are going to lie down and lift your upper body off the floor, making it part of the resistance your core muscles have to work against. Talk about challenging—you will feel all the abdominal muscles after just a few repetitions of this exercise, and you'll be asking for more.

Preparation

1. Lie on your back on either an exercise mat or a carpeted surface. Bend your knees until your feet are about 1 foot from your butt. Keep your feet flat on the floor.

2. Hold a medicine ball of the appropriate size and weight for your ability level in both hands directly above your head and shoulders.

3. Keep your arms straight. Perform a crunch, lifting your head and shoulders off the floor. Hold this position.

Movement

4. Rotate your body to one side until you can almost touch the ball to the floor next to you. You may have to crunch up a little farther to keep your shoulders off the floor.

5. Rotate back to the starting position and on over to the other side, reaching the ball toward the floor next to you again.

6. Continue rotating left and right for 10 repetitions on each side, while keeping your shoulders from touching back down.

7. Rest for 15–20 seconds before beginning your second and third sets.

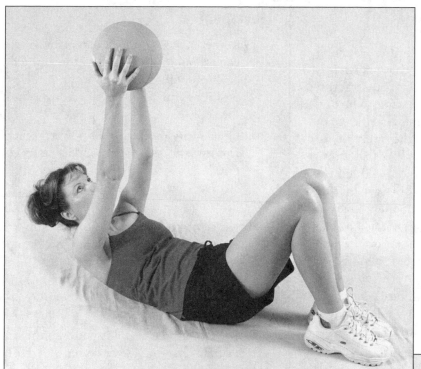

Starting/ending position.

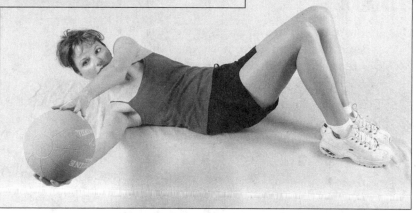

Midpoint position.

Rocky Abs

I stole the idea for this exercise after watching reruns of old *Rocky* movies. In these movies, there is always a scene of Rocky Balboa getting ready for a big fight, doing all kinds of boxing exercises, running, and abdominal work. They didn't know it then, but what they were doing was core conditioning. Don't think that after doing this exercise you can go out and fight some "unbeatable" heavyweight—save that for later. This exercise adds a component of speed to a bit of the lying Russian twist. You'll do this exercise for time instead of repetitions because as you get stronger, you will get faster—so judge your improvement by how many repetitions you can get done in a minute (assuming that you are able to do this for a full minute—gee, was that a challenge, champ?).

Preparation

1. Lie on your back on an exercise mat or a carpeted surface. Bend your knees so that your feet are no more than a foot away from your butt.

2. Hold a medicine ball against your chest, just under your chin. Keep one hand on each side of the ball, and keep your elbows tight against your sides.

Movement

3. Roll your head and shoulders up until your shoulder blades don't touch the floor anymore. Hold your abs tight in this position; you don't get to go down until the set is over.

4. Quickly and with a lot of power, rotate from side to side as fast and as far as you can. You may have to crunch up a little farther to keep your shoulders from touching the floor.

5. Keep rotating back and forth for up to a minute. When you can do a full minute, count how many reps you get (left is one, right is two, left is three, and so on) in a minute. Then concentrate on going faster and getting more reps every minute.

6. Rest for 15–20 seconds between the three or four sets you'll love doing.

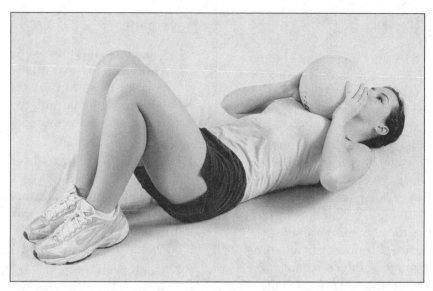

Starting/ending position.

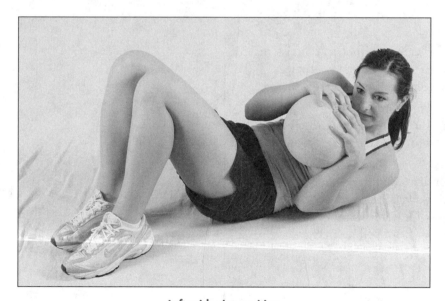

Left midpoint position.

Lying Hip Roll

We are going to try something a little different now and let your lower body do the rotating while your upper body stays still. With the lying hip rolls, your upper body has to stabilize and keep you from just rolling over on your side, while your lower body has to work against the weight of your legs plus the weight of the medicine ball. You'll feel this exercise a little differently than the others so far because the core muscles will be working but your trunk won't move. This causes the abdominals and lower back to both stabilize the movement and provide some of the motion at the same time. It's an interesting feeling that will provoke your core to strengthen in a whole new way.

Preparation

1. Lie on your back on either an exercise mat or a carpeted surface. Bend your knees until your feet are about 2 feet from your butt, a little farther away than normal.

2. Place your medicine ball between your knees, and squeeze your knees together to hold it there.

3. Place your arms and hands out to your sides, with your palms pressed against the floor to provide some additional stability and keep you from rolling over.

Movement

4. Keep the ball squeezed between your knees, and twist your lower body to bring your knees down toward the floor on your left side. You may not get your knees all the way to the floor; that's okay—you will in time.

5. When you are rotated as far to the left as you can, bring your knees back up to the starting position and rotate them over to the right as far as you can. While you are twisting from side to side, your feet should stay on the floor.

6. Continue rotating left and right until you have finished 20 repetitions. Rest for 15–20 seconds before starting the next set.

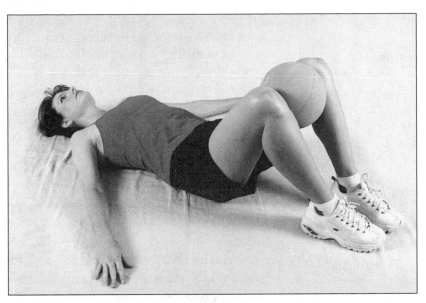

Starting/ending position.

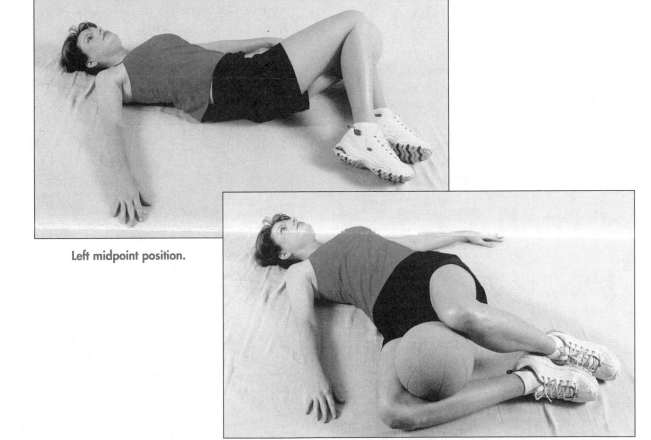

Left midpoint position.

Right midpoint position.

Pendulum

Picture a pendulum swinging from side to side. Got it? That's exactly what you are going to do in this exercise. In real life, a pendulum swings from side to side, slowly losing energy and moving less each time. You, on the other hand, are only going to get better each swing, gaining energy and moving more. During this exercise, the muscles in the lower back and glutes are going to be stabilizing your upper body to keep you from falling forward, while the core abdominals will do most of the work moving you from side to side. It's actually a very relaxing exercise for the first few reps, and then it becomes challenging.

Preparation

1. Stand with your feet shoulder-width apart, knees slightly bent.

2. Hold a medicine ball of the appropriate size and weight for your ability in both hands, with one hand on each side of the ball. Hold the ball down in front of you.

3. Bend at the waist as far as you can without bending your knees anymore or falling over. Let your arms and the ball hang down toward the ground in a relaxed position. Keep your back as straight as you can.

Movement

4. Slowly rotate your body to one side, bringing the ball up and out to your side as far as you can while keeping your back straight.

5. Let gravity take over and bring you back down to the starting position and on across toward the other side (like a pendulum swinging). Use your abdominal and lower-back muscles to help the ball up and out to that side as far as you can rotate.

6. Continue "swinging" from side to side, each time trying to rotate as far as possible, until you complete all 20 repetitions. Rest 15–20 seconds; then do two more sets.

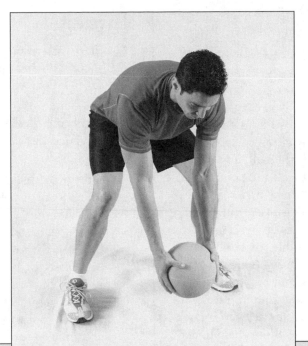

Starting/ending position.

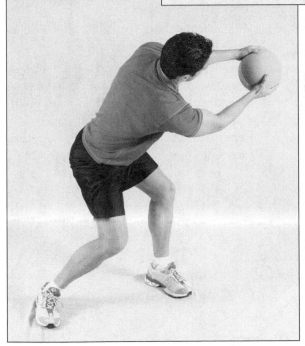

Left midpoint position.

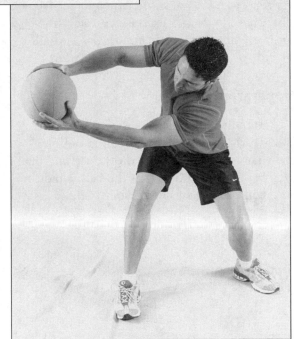

Right midpoint position.

Cross-Throw

Now it's time to get a buddy involved again. You'll need a partner for the next three exercises. If your partner wants to do these exercises as well, that would be perfect—you can throw back and forth and both get your workout done. The cross-throw uses mostly rotation to produce the force needed to throw the ball. You won't throw it very far, but that isn't the point anyway, unless you're one of those hyperaggressive competitive types—in which case, bring it on! As long as your core muscles contract and produce as much force as possible, that's all that matters. Use a ball that is heavy enough for you to feel while you work, but not so heavy that you have a hard time holding it up in place. This exercise challenges your core muscles to rotate quickly and then release, teaching them to act and relax as fast as possible. You will need some space to do this exercise correctly and not break anything when you throw the ball. Outside or on a basketball court is perfect.

Preparation

1. Stand with your feet shoulder-width apart. Hold a medicine ball in both hands, with one hand on the top and one hand on the bottom of the ball. Hold the ball out to one side of your body.

Movement

2. Start with a small, quick backward movement to "wind up" your torso a little more before you throw.

3. Rebound out of the backward movement, and bring the ball out and across in front of you as fast as you can. Keep your arms straight, and keep a good grip on the ball.

4. Throw the ball out to your side using as much force as you can. Try not to push the ball with one hand more than the other; your goal is to let go of the ball with both hands at the same time. You should aim to release the ball just as it passes directly in front of you. If you release it much past this point, it will land more behind you than out to your side. Let your body continue to rotate around in a "follow-through" motion.

5. Your partner should stand to your side to catch the ball.

6. Have your partner catch the ball and toss it back to you. Complete a set of 10 throws from one side; then switch and complete a set of 10 throws from the other side. Repeat this again for a total of two sets on each side.

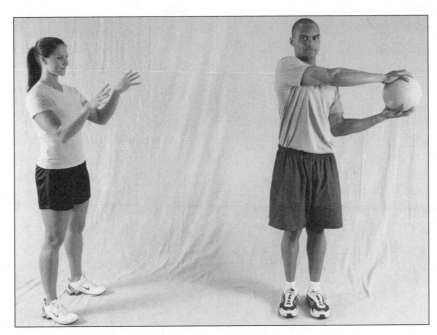

Starting/ending position.

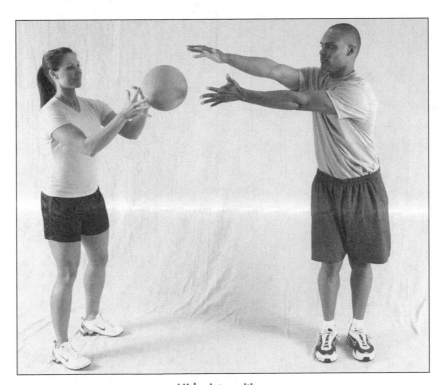

Midpoint position.

Diagonal Throw

The diagonal throw is similar to the cross-throw, except that now you get to include some of the glutes and hip extensor muscles, along with more shoulder involvement, to get the ball moving faster and to throw it farther. Because you will be throwing the ball up and out, you should do this exercise outside or in a gymnasium— somewhere with a high ceiling and nothing nearby that can get broken. If you want to really sound like you are working as hard as it looks, grunt a little when you let go of the ball.

Preparation

1. Stand with your feet shoulder-width apart. Bend your knees and hips until you are in about a half-squat position.

2. Hold the ball out to one side, somewhere between your knees and ankles, but not touching the floor.

Movement

3. Start with a small, quick backward movement to "wind up" your torso a little more before you throw.

4. Rebound out of the backward movement, and bring the ball up and across in front of you as fast as you can. Keep your arms straight, and keep a good grip on the ball.

5. Release the ball when it is just past your midsection. When you release the ball, let go with both hands at the same time. Don't let one hand push the ball more than the other. This isn't an arm exercise; the core muscles are providing the force through their quick rotation. The ball should move up and out to the side of your body. Because of the upward trajectory, the ball will travel farther and build up more momentum than during the cross-throw.

6. Have your partner catch the ball and toss it back to you. Repeat 10 throws to one side and then 10 throws from the other side for one set. Rest a minute and do another set.

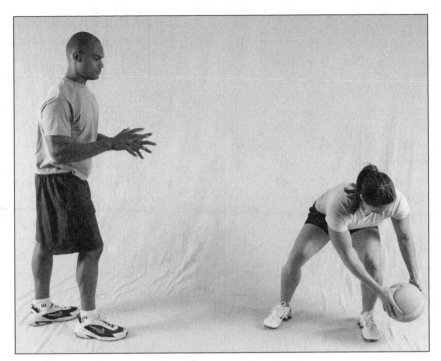

Starting/ending position.

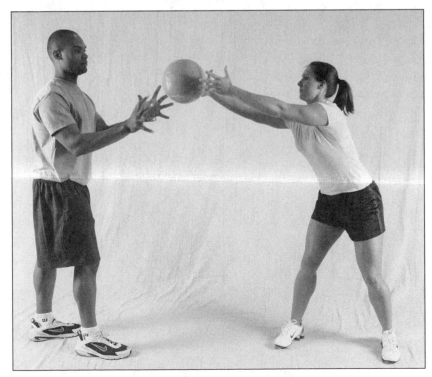

Midpoint position.

Overhead Throw

The overhead throw doesn't involve any rotation, but your core muscles are still going to do most of the work. In this exercise, the core abdominals provide the force to throw the ball. There is some work done by the shoulders and upper-back muscles, but we want to minimize that as much as possible. When you do this correctly, you won't move a whole lot, but the ball will fly through the air. You and your partner can actually throw the ball back and forth, kind of like a game of keep-away.

Preparation

1. Stand with your feet shoulder-width apart. Hold the appropriate size and weight of medicine ball for your ability over your head, with your arms straight. Keep one hand on each side of the ball.

Movement

2. Start with a small, quick backward movement to "wind up" your torso a little more before you throw.

3. Rebound out of the wind-up quickly, and flex your abdominal muscles to bring the ball forward. Release the ball before you start to push it with your arms. The goal is to produce all the force with your core, not your arms. You won't throw the ball very far. When you let go of the ball, your arms should still be above your head.

4. Have your partner catch the ball and throw it back to you so that you catch it over your head.

5. Allow the momentum of the ball to carry you back into your wind-up position. Rebound out of this and throw the ball again. Repeat until you finish 15 repetitions in each of three sets.

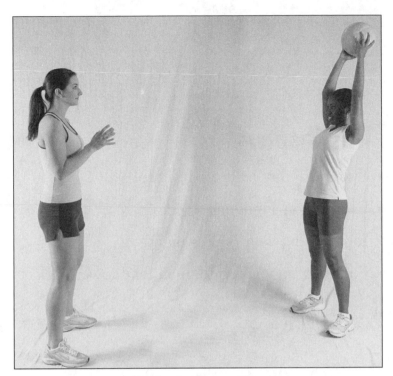

Starting/ending position.

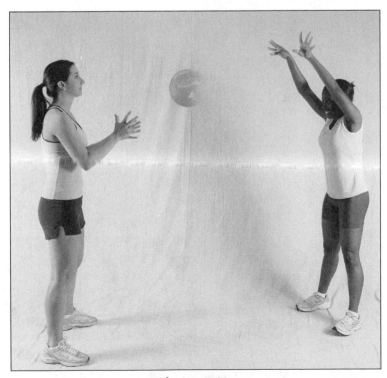

Midpoint position.

In This Chapter

- ◆ Using stability balls for leverage
- ◆ Exercise on a moving object
- ◆ Intensifying your body weight
- ◆ Focusing on your abdominals and lower back

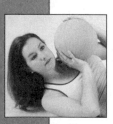
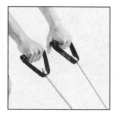
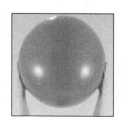
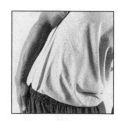
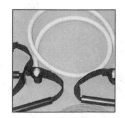
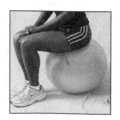

Chapter 10

Beginning Stability Ball Exercises

Back in the early 1970s, a couple of physical therapists wondered what would happen if they had a patient exercise while sitting on a big ball instead of a bench or chair. So they found an oversize playground ball and brought it to work. Soon patients were sitting, lying, and bouncing around on the balls all over the office. Other than it just being fun, the therapists noticed that their patients were progressing through their rehab programs faster than ever, and leaving in better shape than they were before they got hurt. Maybe they were on to something?

It took another 20 years for the mainstream fitness communities to latch on to the idea that stability balls, then called Swiss balls, could provide another level of intensity to a normal person's workout. Over the last 10 years, stability balls have become part of every fitness center's equipment lineup and can now be purchased at just about any sporting goods store (although the quality can vary—see Appendix B for good sources). This chapter introduces you to the stability ball and how you can incorporate it into your core-conditioning program with ease. It's really just a tool that takes away the solid surface of the floor you are used to lying or sitting on, gives you some additional leverage, and allows you to move through some wider ranges of motion than your body is used to. This gives you another advantage in the fight against a sagging core and the means to change up your workout in yet another direction.

Ball Crunch

Probably the oldest use of the stability ball is the ball crunch. The idea behind this exercise is that if you take away the solid floor a person is used to working on and make the surface unstable, that person will have to engage more of the core muscles to keep in the correct position (and not fall off). It actually works exactly as described. When you do ball crunches, you will notice that your hips will tend to drift from side to side, and your hip and butt muscles will be working to help keep you on top of the ball. In addition to all that, you can move through a larger range of motion, giving you greater results than a normal crunch. This is probably one of the easiest stability ball exercises, but it's a foundation exercise that you should master before moving on to other, more difficult stability ball movements. It's time to lie down and wiggle around!

Preparation

1. Sit on top of the appropriate size of stability ball for your height (see Chapter 3 for correct sizing). Keep your feet together in front of you.

2. Slowly walk your feet out from the ball, and lie back on the ball. Stop when the top of the ball is in the curve of your lower back.

3. Cross your arms across your chest, with your fingers touching your shoulders.

4. Let your back relax around the curve of the ball (you will be bent over backward just a little bit).

Movement

5. Take a deep breath in. As you exhale, slowly roll your head, shoulders, and chest up off the ball until only your lower back is touching and you can see straight out in front of you.

6. Breathe in as you lower yourself back to the starting point and begin another repetition. Complete 30 repetitions in each of three sets. Rest for 15–20 seconds between each set.

Variations

If you have trouble keeping your hips under you while you crunch (the ball moves around a lot), spread your feet wider apart until you feel more stable. Any exercise on a stability ball is less stable with your feet close together because your base of support is smaller, and more stable with your feet wide apart where your base of support is very large.

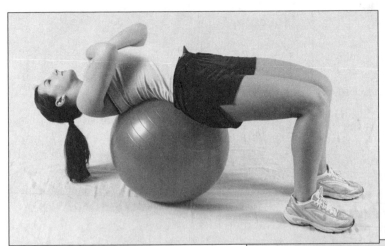

Starting/ending position.

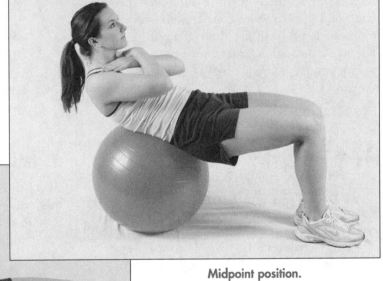

Midpoint position.

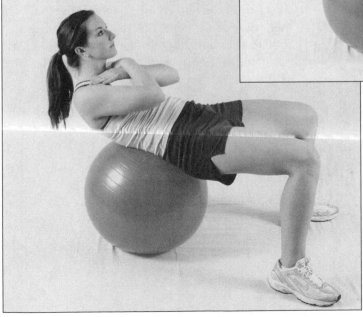

Variation with feet wider apart.

Ball Oblique

Ball obliques are a little more challenging than ball crunches. This exercise seeks to target the same muscles as oblique crunches do: the core abdominals and internal/external obliques. What makes ball obliques a bit tougher is the way your body moves over the ball. When you twist your torso during this exercise, you will be pushing on one side of the ball a bit more than the other, making the ball try to squeeze out from under you. Your core hip and glute muscles will work to help keep the ball in place, so you will definitely feel the difference from lying on the floor. Your core abdominals and oblique muscles will fire more than usual as you work through a larger range of motion, giving you larger-than-usual benefits.

Preparation

1. Sit on top of the appropriate size of stability ball for your height (see Chapter 3 for correct sizing). Keep your feet together in front of you.

2. Slowly walk your feet out from the ball, and lie back on the ball. Stop when the top of the ball is in the curve of your lower back.

3. Cross your arms across your chest, with your fingers touching your shoulders.

4. Let your back relax around the curve of the ball (you will be bent over backward just a little bit).

Movement

5. Starting with either the left or right shoulder, slowly roll your head and one shoulder up off the ball. As you roll up, breathe out and bring that shoulder across your body, aiming it for the opposite foot (left shoulder toward right foot, right shoulder toward left foot). The other shoulder will come up off the ball a little bit but should not rotate across the body. It will actually move down toward the ball as the other shoulder crosses over.

6. Return to the starting position, take a deep breath in, and repeat to the other side.

7. Continue alternating from left to right until you have completed 30 repetitions. Do three sets, resting about a minute between each one.

Variations

If you find the ball trying to scoot out from under you, or if your hips tend to move from side to side, spread your feet a little wider apart until you feel more stable and comfortable.

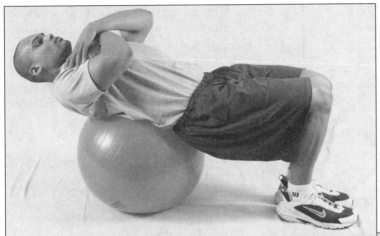

Starting/ending position.

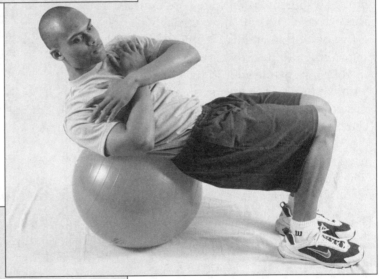

Midpoint position.

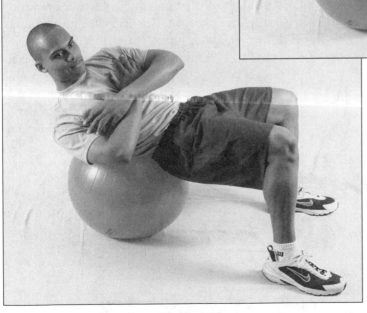

Variation with feet wider apart.

Glute Ham Raise

A benefit of using a stability ball is that you can target muscles that you can't really get without big, expensive machines. A perfect example is the glute ham raise. This exercise goes after the big muscles of your glutes and hamstrings, and the smaller muscles of your lower back and deep posterior. Although the hamstrings are not typically considered part of your core because they are in your legs, the origin of these muscles overlaps with several of the core muscles, and they affect movement at your hips—so sometimes they are core muscles. In this exercise, you will move through a large range of motion and feel the muscles in your butt tighten to provide movement and stability of your hips, while your lower back will roll up with the help of the erector spinae and deep posterior muscles. That's a lot of muscles being activated at one time, and all from a little exercise on a big ball. For this exercise, you will need to anchor your feet at the base of a wall. The best wall is one made of brick, rock, or wood. If you are doing this in your home, you may scuff the paint on a normal wall, so close a solid door and use that instead.

Preparation

1. Anchor your feet by setting your toes on the floor and your heels against the wall. Keep your legs straight.

2. Lie face down over your ball. Position the ball so that the top of it is at your waist, and you can lie over the top of the ball so your head is lower than your hips.

3. Relax over the ball, letting all your muscles loosen and stretch. Cross your arms over your chest, with your fingers touching your shoulders.

Movement

4. Take a deep breath in. As you blow it out, roll your back up until your body is straight, and continue to tighten your back and butt muscles until you have lifted your upper body. Your upper legs and hips will stay on the ball.

5. Slowly lower yourself back to the starting position. Do 10–15 repetitions to complete the set. Rest for 15–20 seconds and do another set.

Precautions

It's important that you not hold your breath during this exercise. Because your head will be lower than your heart, you may experience a "head rush" sensation as you perform this exercise. If you do, stop until it passes and continue with the exercise while breathing deeply with each repetition. If the sensation does not pass and you feel dizzy, discontinue this exercise until you consult with your doctor.

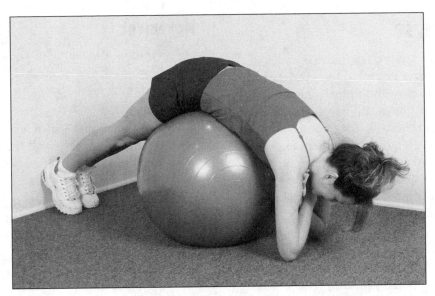

Starting/ending position.

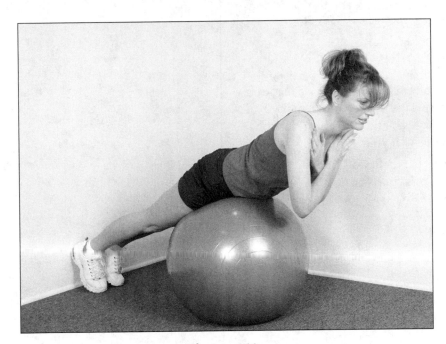

Midpoint position.

Ball Reverse

The ball reverse adds a few more muscles to the normal reverse crunch. Here, you will be focusing on the core abdominals, but at the same time, your glutes and hamstrings will be working to hold the ball. Your abdominals then have to work even harder because some of the muscles that oppose the abdominals are working. Think of it like pushing a shopping cart. If you are just pushing it, it's easy; but if someone is pushing back, you have to work harder to move forward. The same principle applies here. When you contract the glutes and hamstrings, the lower back tightens a little bit (just like during the glute ham raise). When the lower back is working, the abdominals have to work harder to contract, so you get more conditioning results.

Preparation

1. Lie on your back on an exercise mat or a carpeted surface. Place your stability ball under your legs, and squeeze it by pushing in on it with your heels.

2. Place your hands flat on the floor at your sides, palms facing down.

Movement

3. Holding the ball with your legs, roll your hips up off the ground. This is easier if you think about bringing your knees toward your chest.

4. Try not to push down with your arms; let your abdominals do all the work. If you feel like you're pushing down, place your hands on your shoulders.

5. When your hips are off the ground, slowly return to the starting position, but do not let the ball touch the ground—keep it squeezed to your legs. Do 20 repetitions to complete your set. Rest a few moments and do another set.

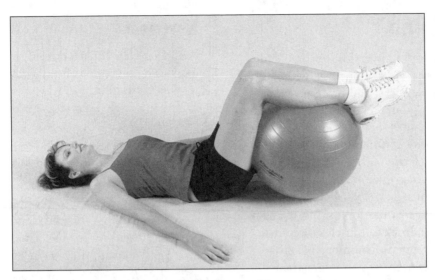

Starting/ending position.

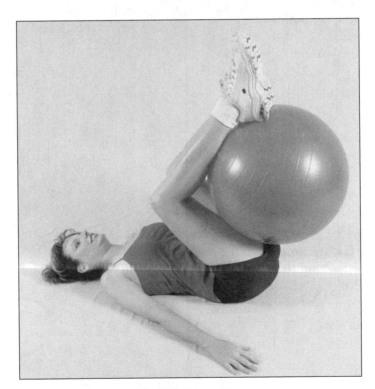

Left midpoint position.

Ball Bridging

You will see a couple of versions of ball bridging in this chapter and the next. As with the body weighted exercises, ball bridging focuses on the muscles in your lower back and glutes. The difference now is that the floor is replaced with a ball that moves when you move. The key here is to keep the ball directly under the shoulders the whole time, not moving from side to side. Because you are going to be up off the floor, the range of motion during the exercise increases to allow the muscles to contract more and longer, giving you more benefits than before. This exercise is tougher than working on the floor. If you need to use your hands to keep from rolling off the sides, you can do that. As you get more comfortable on the ball, keep your hands across your chest or at your waist, and let your core muscles hold you in place.

Preparation

1. Sit on top of your ball, with your feet together in front of you.

2. If you are still getting the hang of this exercise, keep your hands down to your sides. If you are feeling comfortable with it, keep your hands across your chest.

3. Slowly walk your feet out away from the ball, allowing your body to slide down and roll off the ball. Stop when your shoulders are the only part of your upper body still touching the ball.

Movement

4. Lift your hips and hold them at the point that your upper body and upper legs are in a straight line. Keep your head back so you are looking at the ceiling.

5. If you need to place your hands on the floor to keep the ball from moving side to side, you can.

6. Hold the bridged position for up to 60 seconds. Return to the starting position by dropping your hips and walking your feet back toward the ball, rolling your body back up into a sitting position.

7. Rest for 15–20 seconds and repeat three more times. Keep increasing the length of each repetition until you can do all four sets for 60 seconds each.

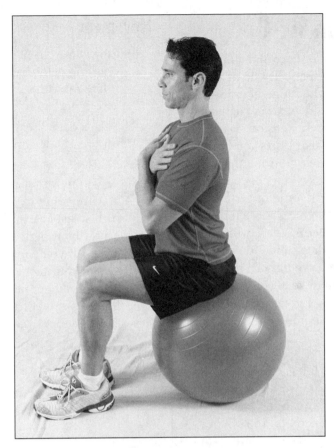

Starting/ending position.

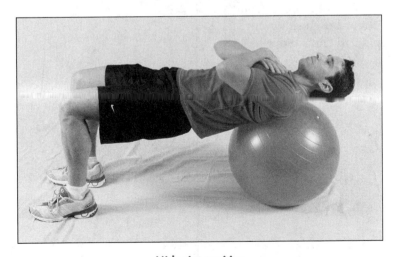

Midpoint position.

Hyperextension Sit-Up

The only way to make your core abdominal muscles work even more than they do in a regular sit-up is to increase the range of motion. Because you can't sit up any further, you have to start farther back. Hyperextension sit-ups do just that. This is a sit-up that starts you from a hyperextended (arched back) position that you can't get on the floor. This results in your core abdominals having to work for a longer period of time, and it actually produces more force than lying on the floor. Because you will be lying on a stability ball, the foundation of your exercise is movable. Your core muscles in the hips and glutes will work to keep you still while you sit up. Overall, this is a great exercise that will really fire up your abdominal muscles.

Preparation

1. Sit on top of your ball, with your feet together in front of you. Slide forward until you are not directly on top of your ball, but just starting to slide down. Hold this position.

2. Hold your arms straight out over your head, pointed toward the ceiling. Interlock your fingers and "hug" your head with your arms.

Movement

3. Slowly lean back until your hands are pointing behind you and down toward the floor. Your upper body should be arched across the top of the ball.

4. Take a deep breath in. As you blow it out, lift your upper body back up to the starting position.

5. As you move up and down, if you feel like you are going to roll off the edge of the ball, adjust and pull yourself back to the center by using your hip muscles and glutes. If you continue to roll off the ball, spread your feet apart until you feel stable. As you get better at this exercise, move your feet back together.

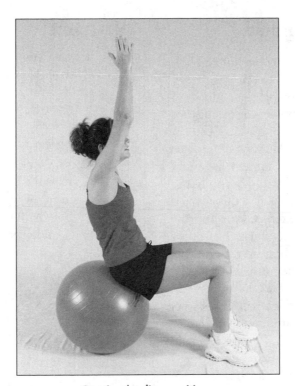

Starting/ending position.

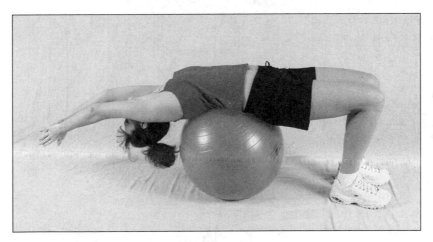

Midpoint position.

Inclined Superman

No, this exercise does not involve flying either. Stop thinking of Superman exercises as flying and think of them as "stronger than a locomotive." The inclined Superman is a stabilization exercise for the lower-back and deep-posterior muscles, as well as the shoulder and upper-back muscles. This exercise takes some work, but the effort you put out now will pay you back in the near future (like tomorrow). I think this is probably one of the best exercises for improving your posture. It's easy to work on sitting up straight in a chair, or standing up straight, but when you make those same muscles do their job while fighting gravity and your upper-body weight, it gets serious. This exercise takes some work to get good at, so start slow and increase your set time until you are at the max; then add more sets to see further improvements. For this exercise, you will need to anchor your feet at the base of a wall. The best wall is made of brick, rock, or wood. If you are doing this in your home, you may scuff the paint on a normal wall, so close a solid door and use that instead.

Preparation

1. Anchor your feet by setting your toes on the floor and your heels against the wall. Keep your legs straight.

2. Lie face down over your ball. Position the ball so that the top of it is at your waist, and you can lie over the top of the ball so your head is lower than your hips.

3. Relax over the ball, letting all your muscles loosen and stretch. Hold your hands straight out over your head in the "flying Superman" position.

Movement

4. Take a deep breath in. As you blow it out, roll your back up until your body is straight, and continue to tighten your back and butt muscles until you have lifted your upper body as high as you can go. Your upper legs and hips will stay on the ball.

5. Continue to point your hands out over your head toward the ceiling. Hold this position for up to 60 seconds. Relax back to the starting position, rest for 15–20 seconds, and repeat for three more sets.

Variations

If you have trouble holding this position without rolling off the top of the ball, spread your feet a little wider to give yourself a bigger foundation.

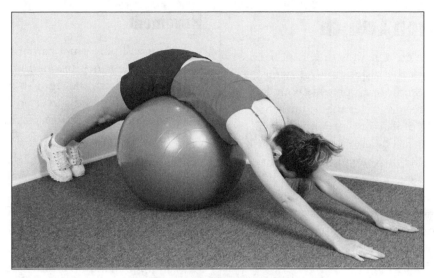

Starting/ending position.

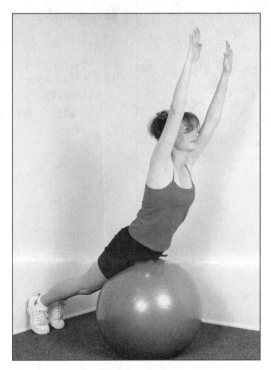

Midpoint position.

Combination Crunch

The combination crunch adds the elements of a ball oblique with the instability of having only one leg on the floor to provide your foundation. This exercise can get shaky, but when you get the hang of it, your core muscles will be in tip-top shape. The core abdominals provide the bulk of the movement, but the hip flexors get into the game with each repetition. What makes this exercise so much fun is that you are constantly switching directions and foot support positions, so each repetition has to be dealt with individually.

Preparation

1. Lie on top of your ball so that the top of the ball is in the curve of your lower back. Let your body arch across the ball.

2. Lift your hips and move your feet away from you. Keep your feet together for maximum instability (it's harder), or move them apart to feel more stable (it's easier).

3. Cross your arms over your chest, with your fingers touching your shoulders.

Movement

4. You will perform a ball oblique and, at the same time, lift one foot off the floor. Starting with the right shoulder, roll the shoulder up and across your body (left shoulder stays down). At the same time, lift your left foot off the ground, pointing your leg out in front of you.

5. Relax back down to the starting position, and repeat by lifting the left shoulder and right leg.

6. Alternate repetitions side to side until you have completed 20 repetitions. Rest a few moments and do another set.

Variations

If lifting your feet keeps you too off-balance, you can repeat to one side for a set, and then do another set to the other side. You can also cross one leg over the other leg and keep your foot in the air for the complete set.

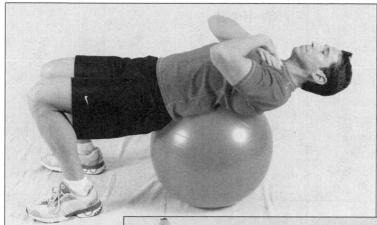

Starting/ending position.

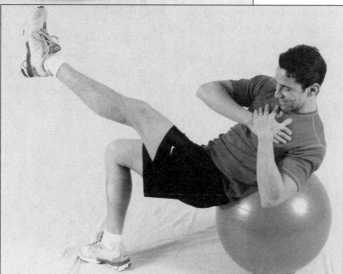

Midpoint position.

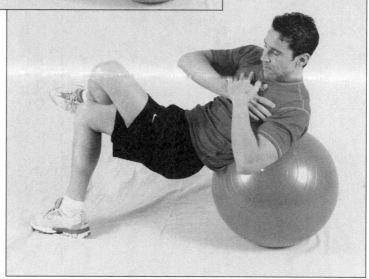

Variation with one leg crossed over the other.

Kneeling Tuck

This exercise shows you how to work your lower back, hip flexors, abdominals, and glutes while facing the floor. Sound strange? It really isn't once you try it. If you did this exercise in any other position, you wouldn't get near the results because the ball allows you to engage quite a few muscles in combination. Kneeling tucks are a favorite of my clients who are getting ready to go skiing. Along with the moguls exercise in the next chapter, the kneeling tuck simulates a motion that is common in downhill skiing, and will help you prepare for that vacation to the mountains.

Preparation

1. Lie face down over your ball.

2. Place your hands on the floor and straighten your arms. Keep your knees and feet together.

3. Slowly "walk" out on your arms until the ball is at your knees. Hold yourself in this position and keep the ball from moving side to side.

Movement

4. While you support your weight with your arms, pull your knees to your chest. To keep the ball from sliding to one side, start slowly until you get the hang of it. You can increase your speed later.

5. Straighten your legs back out and do this exercise for 10–15 repetitions. Rest for a minute and do two more sets.

Variations

You can make this exercise even more difficult if you keep one leg straight and bend only one knee at a time. This puts all the stabilization on one side of your body while the other side is holding the nonmoving leg in the air.

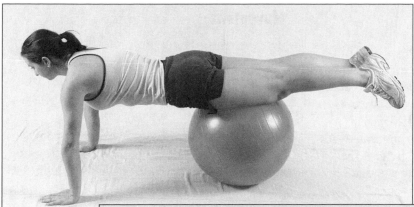

Starting/ending position.

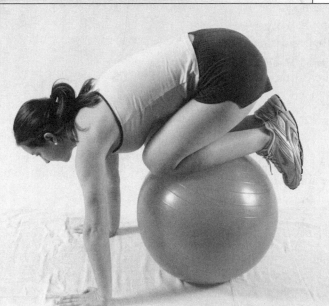

Midpoint position.

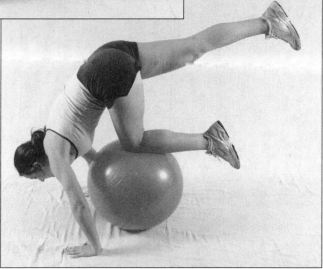

Variation with one leg straight.

Touchdown

I had to get you standing for at least one exercise in this chapter—don't want you getting a little too used to lying down and begin to doze off. Touchdowns bring your whole body into play. You will be moving your entire core, including the muscles in the legs and arms—it's an all-over exercise. This one really gets the blood pumping and is a great way to wake up in the morning. A couple sets of touchdowns, and there is no going back to sleep. The touchdown could be a medicine ball exercise, but it's designed to get you moving through a range of motion without providing a lot of resistance. We haven't had much rotation in this chapter, so here it comes.

Preparation

1. Stand with your feet about shoulder-width apart. Hold your stability ball over your head, with one hand on each side of the ball and your arms straight.

Movement

2. Bring the stability ball down and out to one side, bending your knees and hips, and rotating so that you touch the ball down behind you as much as possible. Return to the starting position.

3. Now go the other way, rotating your body in the opposite direction. Continue alternating touchdowns left and right for a total of 30 repetitions. Complete two more sets, resting about 15 seconds between sets.

Variations

For more intensity, bend your knees and hips more and increase your speed. Make sure you stand all the way up and stretch your arms high between each repetition. (I told you this could really get your blood pumping!)

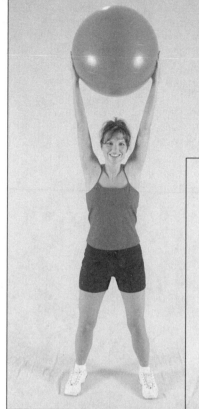

Starting/ending position.

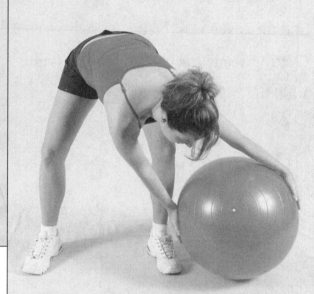

Left midpoint position.

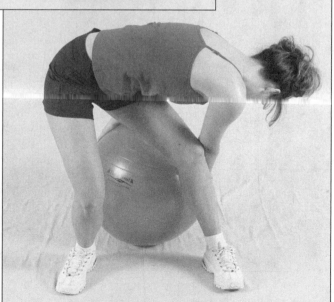

Variation with knees bent more.

In This Chapter

- ◆ Building unstable bridges

- ◆ Stability exercises for the legs

- ◆ Getting ready for black diamond skiing

- ◆ Walking on your hands

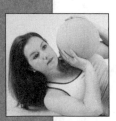
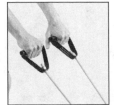
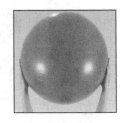
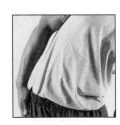
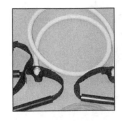
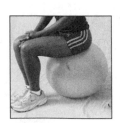

11

Advanced Stability Ball Exercises

There are countless ways you can use a stability ball, some of them passive and easy, some more difficult. Because you want a solid core, passive and easy doesn't cut it. This chapter takes stability ball exercises one step further, placing more stress on the legs without actually using the leg muscles very much. The stress all comes from the core—specifically, the hip flexors, rotators, and extensors. These are still muscles you can't see much of. The big glute muscles will be working, and you can touch those if you like, but the really good muscles are deep down next to your bones. These short, powerful muscles have only one job to do: keep your legs where they are supposed to be. That's no easy job because your legs are usually in motion, and not always with you in complete control. Core conditioning allows you to take control and move in a purposeful and meaningful way. The goal is to make movement more fluid and graceful, like a ballet dancer. But don't put on those dance slippers just yet—you'll need those cross-training shoes for this chapter.

This chapter also involves a lot of balance exercises, designed to make your core muscles contract and hold in place. This gives you more "time under tension," a term that means the muscle is working for a long time—the longer, the better. Make sure you have mastered the beginning stability ball exercises in the previous chapter before tackling these.

Hang on and have fun!

Back Bridge

You've done several variations of the bridge so far, but this exercise takes the cake. The most difficult of all the bridging exercises makes your core hip muscles do a ton of work because your feet are no longer on solid ground. Back bridges introduce a new level of stabilization, from the ground up. When the foundation you are pushing against moves, your body has to move to react and keep you from falling over. That's a big job for a bunch of little muscles. The hip rotators will be working alongside the lower back and deep posteriors, abdominals, and hamstrings. You may feel this one in the hamstrings more than anywhere else because these big muscles aren't being allowed to move and they don't like it. Resist the temptation to give in on this exercise. It takes a while to get good at it, but with patience and practice, all this bridging will get you to a place you never knew existed: fitness from the inside out.

Preparation

1. Lie on your back on an exercise mat or a carpeted surface.

2. Keep your knees bent, and place your feet on top of your stability ball. Try to keep your feet flat against the ball.

3. Place your hands down at your sides, palms facing the floor. When you get good at this exercise, place your arms across your chest to increase the stabilizing effect.

Movement

4. Press on the ball with your feet, lifting your hips up into the air until your body is in a straight line from your knees to your shoulders.

5. Hold this position for up to 60 seconds.

6. Relax back to the floor and rest for 15–20 seconds. Do three more sets.

Precautions

If you feel any pain in your neck or cramping in your back or hamstrings, stop immediately and rest. Pain in the neck or back should be described to your doctor before you continue.

Variations

You can make this exercise even more difficult by using only one foot. Hold one foot up in the air, and press against the ball with the other. To do this correctly and not roll off the side of the ball, keep the foot you are using in the middle of the ball (right on top).

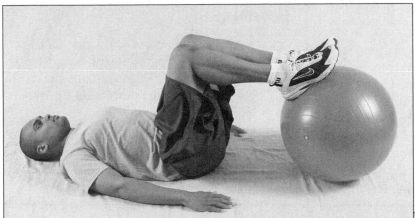

Starting/ending position.

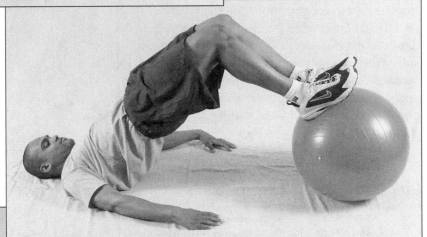

Midpoint position.

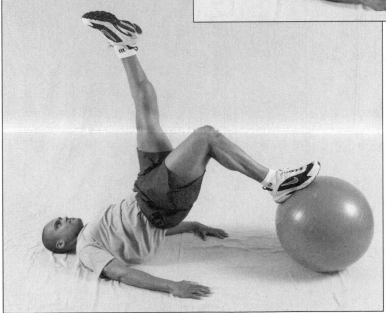

Variation with one foot on the ball.

Pike

A pike is defined by the dictionary as a long stick with a pointed end, used in medieval times as a weapon—kind of like a big pointed stick. This exercise won't make you a knight in shining armor, but it will make you a fit person with a solid core—and that's much better (unless you are a damsel in distress who needs saving from the tower). *Pike* is a word used to describe the position you are moving into during this exercise. The movement comes solely from the hip flexors. These are small muscles that you can actually feel part of in the crease of your hip. Their job is to lift your knee toward your chest, such as when you take a step forward and don't want to drag your toe on the ground. This exercise strengthens the hip flexors and also the core abdominals and lower back that work to stabilize the upper body while you move your legs—it's all tied together.

Preparation

1. Lie on the floor on an exercise mat or a carpeted surface. Prop yourself up on your elbows.

2. Place your stability ball between your feet, using one foot on each side to hold it in place.

3. Use your abdominal muscles to keep your torso straight from your hips to your shoulders—no sagging your back toward the floor.

Movement

4. Keep your upper body straight and still. Lift the ball using both legs. Keep your legs straight as you lift the ball as high as you can—up to the point right over your hips.

5. Slowly lower the ball back down, but don't let it touch the ground. When it gets close (within an inch) of the floor, lift it back up again. Repeat this 10–15 times for your first set, rest a few moments, and repeat for two more sets.

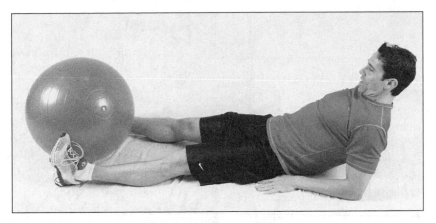

Starting/ending position.

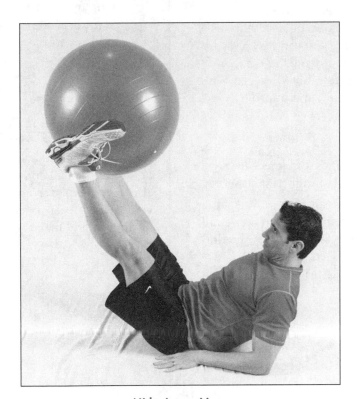

Midpoint position.

Walkout

No, this doesn't mean you get to leave your job or this exercise session. In this case, a walkout is done with your hands. This exercise tests your ability to keep your body straight while your arms are moving and the foundation gets more wobbly. The core abdominals and lower back are really working with this movement, especially the lower back. It's easy to let your body sag like an old horse, but that defeats the purpose. After a few weeks of this exercise, you will notice a marked improvement in your posture, especially when you are sitting down (especially if you are sitting on a stability ball). As you get good at this, you can play around with how you move your hands to make it more challenging and fun, but always in ways that make your core work and improve.

Preparation

1. Kneel on your hands and knees over your stability ball, the ball tight against your stomach.
2. Keep your knees and feet together at all times. Your hands should be on the floor, shoulder-width apart.

Movement

3. Holding yourself up on your arms and hands, slowly "walk out" from the ball on your hands. It's just like the wheelbarrow races you did as a kid, with someone holding your legs while you walked on your hands. This time the ball is holding your legs, but it's not stable. Keep your body in a straight line from the shoulders to the ankles—no sagging.
4. Walk out until the ball is at your shins (or ankles, for more work); then change directions and walk back in until the ball is at your waist. Repeat walkouts to the ankles and back to the waist.

Variations

Of course, you can make this exercise more difficult. Cross one leg over the other so only one leg is touching the ball. Keep that leg directly on top of the ball and do your walkouts. You can also alter the pattern of your hands. Keeping your hands closer together decreases your base of support and makes it more challenging.

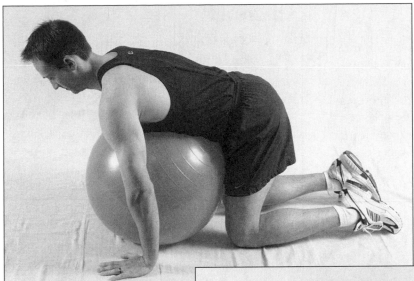

Starting/ending position.

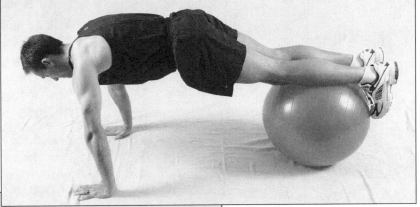

Midpoint position.

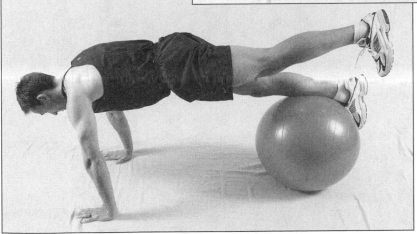

Variation with one leg touching the ball.

Walkout and Point

We can change the regular walkout into more of a stabilization exercise if we decrease the number of balance points you have. What's that? Three balance points is already too few? I say that unless you have only one balance point left, there's always room to make it more fun. In the walkout and point, you perform the same walkout, but instead of just moving back and forth, you hold the walkout position and balance. This makes the core muscles work during the movement, increase their time under tension, and really fire up to keep you from twisting and falling to the floor (it's not that far down anyway).

Preparation

1. Kneel on your hands and knees over your stability ball; the ball should be tight against your stomach.

2. Keep your knees and feet together at all times. Your hands should be on the floor, shoulder-width apart.

Movement

3. While holding yourself up on your arms and hands, slowly "walk out" from the ball on your hands. Keep your body in a straight line from the shoulders to the ankles—no sagging or swaying from side to side.

4. Walk out until the ball is at your shins or ankles.

5. Stop and lift one arm, and point directly in front of you. Hold this position, balanced on one hand, for up to 60 seconds.

6. Put your hand down, lift the other hand, and point directly in front of you. Hold this position for up to 60 seconds.

7. Put your hand down and walk back in. Rest for 15–20 seconds and repeat for three more sets.

Variations

You can make this more challenging by crossing one leg over the other and balancing on just one arm and one leg.

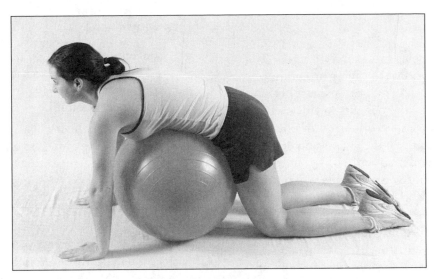

Starting/ending position.

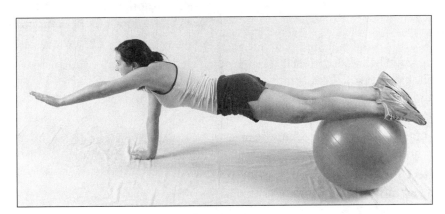

Midpoint position.

Glute Lift

Guess which muscles this exercise targets? If you said glutes, you were paying attention to the title—very smart you are. A smart person will also recognize the benefits of this exercise. My female clients especially love this one because it targets the butt. When you do this exercise consistently, not only will your core be in better shape, but your backside will become more firm. Don't be fooled into thinking this is easy. While you are focusing on your glutes, your lower back is doing the majority of the work. Once you start this exercise, you'll see what I mean. That lower back has to hold up and move your entire lower body—not a job it was designed for, but a heck of an exercise.

Preparation

1. Kneel facing your ball. Let yourself lie over the ball, placing your hands in front of you shoulder-width apart. Keep the ball right under your thighs.

2. Hold your upper body straight from the hips to the shoulders.

3. Keep your feet together, with your legs straight out behind the ball, just a few inches off the floor.

Movement

4. Concentrate on tightening the buttocks and lifting your legs as high as you can. Keep your legs straight and really squeeze the glutes as you lift.

5. Slowly lower the legs back toward the floor, relax the glutes, and then do another 10–15 repetitions. Rest a few moments and do two more sets.

Precautions

Make sure you do this exercise slowly and under control. Don't try to jerk your legs off the floor quickly because that can cause your back to tighten and spasm. Lift and lower your legs in a smooth, deliberate motion.

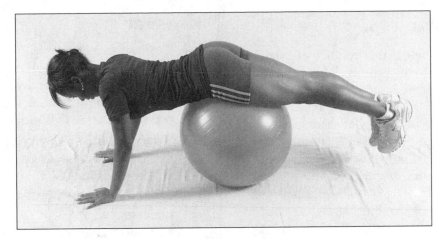

Starting/ending position.

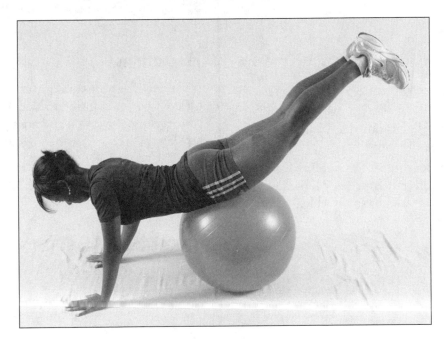

Midpoint position.

Leg Twist

It's time to do the twist! If you like that dance from the '50s, this exercise is right up your alley. But even if you don't normally do the twist, this exercise can help with agility and during such activities as roller skating and skiing. Leg twists target the hip rotators. For once, the core abdominal and lower-back muscles get to rest (this may become one of your favorite exercises). Leg twists seem simple at first glance, but controlling the stability ball and increasing your speed make them a challenging workout.

Preparation

1. Lie on your back on an exercise mat or a carpeted surface. Place your stability ball between your feet, with one foot on each side.

2. Place your hands down at your sides, palms pressing into the floor.

3. Use your legs to lift the stability ball up in the air directly over your hips. Keep your legs as straight as possible.

Movement

4. Begin by turning the ball clockwise as far as you can by using your hips and legs. As you twist, your feet have to stay in contact with the ball, or you'll drop it. Keep pressing into the ball with both feet.

5. When you have rotated clockwise as far as you can, reverse directions and rotate counterclockwise as far as possible.

6. Continue rotating back and forth while increasing your speed. Each left and right movement counts as one repetition. Do 30 repetitions in each of three sets, with about a minute of rest between each set.

Precautions

If you feel your hips and lower back start to lift off the floor or roll side to side, you are getting your torso too involved and are not letting your hips do the work. Slow down a little until you are moving only your legs.

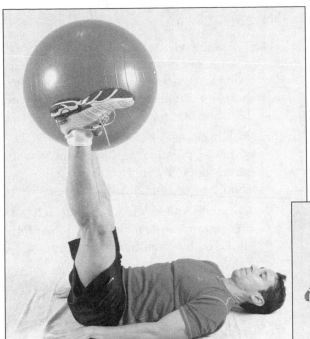

Starting/ending position.

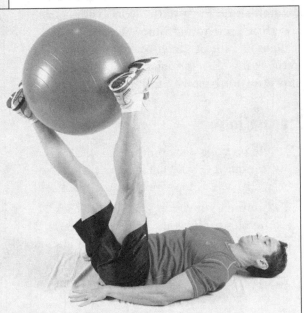

Clockwise midpoint position.

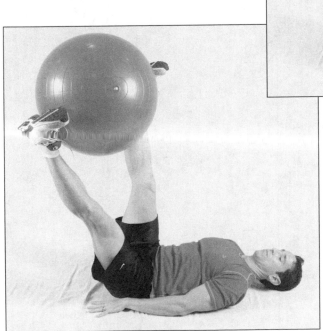

Counterclockwise midpoint position.

Russian Ball Twist

The Russian ball twist tests your ability to move across the top of the ball without falling off the sides of it. Don't worry, though—even if you do fall off the side, you're only about a foot off the ground and are not moving very fast, so it will be more funny than painful. This exercise challenges your lower core muscles and legs to keep you on the ball, while your upper body moves from side to side. Your core abdominals do most of the work, with your lower back providing some stability. There really isn't a lot of carryover from this exercise to the real world, but it's a lot of fun and will improve your balance on the ball.

Preparation

1. Lie on your back on the ball. Walk your feet out until the ball is in the middle of your back. Keep your feet together.

2. Contract your glutes and lower-back muscles to lift your hips so that your body is in a straight line from your shoulders to your knees.

3. Clasp your hands together and point your arms toward the ceiling.

Movement

4. Keeping your feet still and your body as straight as possible, roll over to your left side until your arms are pointing to your left. You should now be balancing on your left shoulder only.

5. Roll back the other way onto your right shoulder, pointing your arms out to your right side. Only your right shoulder should be touching the ball now.

6. Continue rolling left and right (each left and right rotation counts as 1 repetition) until you have finished 30 repetitions.

7. Relax for 15–20 seconds, and then do two more sets.

Variations

To make this twist a little harder and even more fun, hold one foot off the ground as you rotate from side to side.

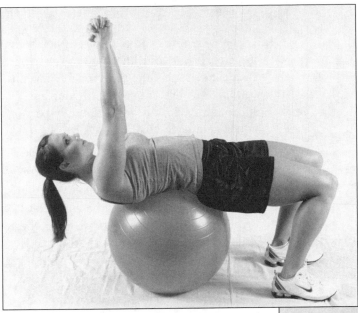

Starting/ending position.

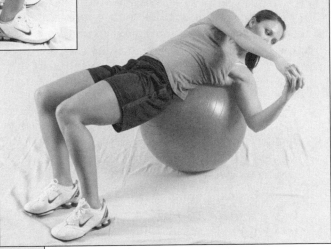

Left midpoint position.

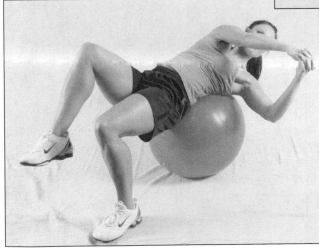

Variation with one foot raised.

Moguls

Moguls are known as the toughest obstacles a skier can face. Part of the reason for this is that skiers must move their lower body independently from their upper body. Sound easy? Well, it isn't—it's a great core challenge. This exercise is similar to the kneeling tuck exercise you learned in Chapter 10, except that instead of bringing your legs straight in, they'll be tucking in and out to the side. This creates rotation in the trunk while the legs come in close to the chest. Just about every muscle in your core is involved in this exercise. Additionally, returning to the starting position in this exercise is a little difficult. You will learn to control your body while it's moving in multiple directions all at once—all part of building a strong core.

Preparation

1. Lie face down over your ball.

2. Place your hands on the floor and straighten your arms. Keep your knees and feet together.

3. Slowly "walk" out on your arms until the ball is at your hips. Hold yourself in this position and keep the ball from moving side to side.

Movement

4. Using your arms to hold your upper body in place, bring your knees up toward your chest, and at the same time rotate your hips so that your legs move out to your left side, and your right leg is the only part of you touching the ball.

5. Straighten back out to the starting position by rolling your legs back under you and straightening them at the same time.

6. Repeat this movement to the right side, bringing your knees up toward your chest and rotating your hips so that the ball is on your right side, and only your left leg is touching the ball.

7. Return to the starting position and continue moguls left and right. One left and one right counts as a single repetition. Continue until you have finished 15 repetitions. Rest for about a minute and do another set.

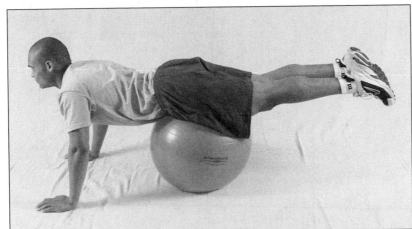

Starting/ending position.

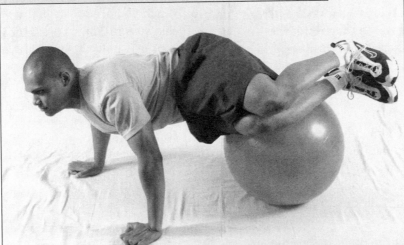

Left midpoint position.

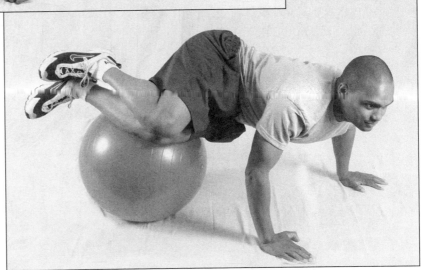

Right midpoint position.

Double Balance

If balance isn't your thing, get ready to make it your thing. When you get the hang of this exercise, you'll be ready for the tightrope (as long as it's on the ground). Up until now, bridging has always involved either your upper or your lower body as a stable point on the ground. Not anymore. In the double balance, your entire body is going to be off the ground, supported by two stability balls. It will take some practice, some more practice, and then a little bit more practice, along with some serious core training, but that is what you're here for. Besides being one of the toughest lower-back and abdominal exercises in this book, it's a great party trick.

Preparation

1. Getting into place for this exercise takes a little bit of manipulation. You'll need two stability balls, preferably the same size. Sit on top of one, and slide down it until the top of the ball is in the middle of your back.

2. Place one foot on the other ball so the ball is under your lower calf. The other foot is still on the floor, keeping you steady.

3. Your hands can begin this exercise down on the floor, helping hold your upper body in place.

4. Lift your hips until your body is in a straight line, with your feet, knees, hips, and shoulders all lined up.

5. Place your other foot on top of the ball next to the first foot. Keep your hands on the floor to steady yourself.

Movement

6. When you are steady and your body is held straight, pick your hands up off the floor and hold them out to your sides (forming a big T).

7. Hold this position for up to 60 seconds, and then relax for 15–20 seconds before the next set. Work up to three sets of 60 seconds each.

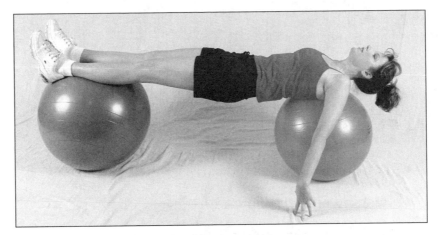

Starting/ending position.

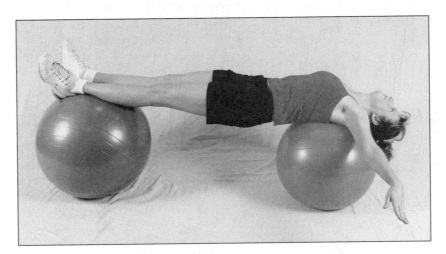

Midpoint position.

In This Chapter

◆ Two forms of resistance are better than one

◆ Pushing and pulling on one leg

◆ Working completely off the ground

◆ How to move and not move at the same time

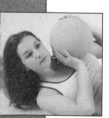 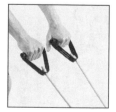 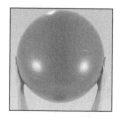 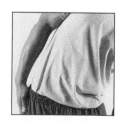 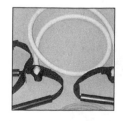 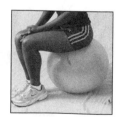

Chapter 12

Multiply the Resistance

If $2 \times 2 = 4$, and $4 \times 4 = 16$, then stability ball $\times$ medicine ball $\times$ resistance tubing $\times$ gravity = a super strong core. Not the simplest math, but the concept is the same. When you use more than one form of resistance and more than one group of core muscles, the result is a greater improvement in core ability and strength than when you train one muscle with one piece of equipment. You don't have to be Einstein to understand the logic in that.

This chapter finishes our journey from the easiest to the most complex core-conditioning exercises. Of course, this isn't every possible exercise you could do, but these are probably some of the most challenging and rewarding of the hundreds available. Some exercises in this chapter will get you totally off the ground, without any source of foundation to stabilize with. By now, you're ready for that. These exercises combine all the elements of balance, power, force, rotation, and movement directions you have conquered, and add a little twist: fun. You won't see these exercises in any magazine; they aren't for everyone—just you guys and gals who have taken the time and put in the effort to make sure that your body is trained from the inside out.

These exercises push your core-conditioning program to a level normally reserved for serious athletes and *Cirque de Soleil* performers. Think of it like this: if you could do one exercise and get the benefits of two or three exercises, wouldn't that be a big time saver? You bet it would. Although they will save you some time, these movements require a bit more skill than you've needed so far. If you have practiced and mastered most of the movements from earlier chapters, then by all means jump right in and get started—you probably need a little more spice in your workout anyway. Your core muscles will definitely notice the difference, and one day you can wow your friends with your core strength and skill.

Seated Ball Toss

When was the last time you threw a ball while sitting down? The answer is probably never. Why not? Well, up until now, we have always been lying down or standing—sitting just doesn't make any sense, which is why we are going to do it. When it doesn't make sense, it makes your muscles really work. The seated ball toss requires a partner who can catch the ball and throw it back to you, preferably someone sitting on a ball just like you and getting a core work-out at the same time. This exercise takes away the stable position you have while standing. The momentum of the ball will have a tendency to try to knock you over backward, so you have to really engage those core muscles to react when you catch the ball and bring it to a stop quickly.

Preparation

1. Sit on the appropriate-sized stability ball for your height (your legs should be paral-lel to the floor, with your hips at the same height as your knees). Keep your feet as close together as you can while staying balanced.

2. Hold a medicine ball that is heavy enough to provide some resistance, but not so heavy that you can't throw it at least 10 feet. Grasp the ball on both sides and hold it under your chin, against your chest.

3. Your partner should stand or sit about 10 feet away from you, ready to receive the ball.

Movement

4. Use both arms and your chest muscles to throw the ball to your partner. When you throw the ball, physics will try to push you backward (for every action, there is an opposite reaction). You have to lean for-ward slightly to keep your balance.

5. Your partner will catch the ball and throw it back to you in the same manner. If your partner throws it correctly, it will come right at your chest.

6. Catch the ball with your arms stretched out in front of you, and absorb the ball's momentum as you bring it in to your chest. Don't let the ball push you over backward. Keep your abdominal and lower-back muscles tight so you are sitting upright at all times.

7. Repeat throwing and catching the ball 20–30 times per set for three sets. Rest about a minute between sets. As you get better at tossing and catching, speed it up so you finish your sets faster.

Precautions

Just to be safe, place an exercise mat behind you, in case you fall over backward during a catch.

Variations

You can increase the amount of balancing you have to do by holding one foot off the ground. This will make you a little more wobbly, but that only heightens the conditioning effect of this exercise.

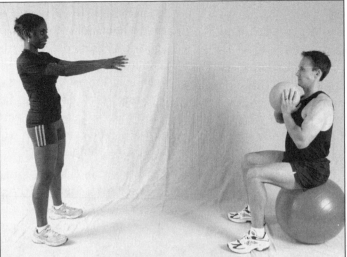

Starting/ending position.

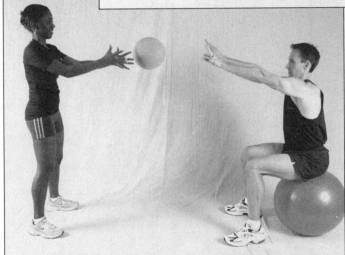

Midpoint position.

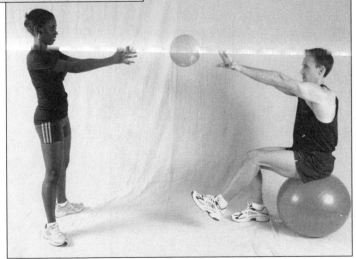

Variation with one foot off the ground.

Bounce Pass

The bounce pass is a derivation of the seated ball toss, with you bouncing the ball to your partner instead of throwing it. The only thing the two exercises have in common is that you will be sitting on a stability ball and your core muscles will be working to the max. Your core muscles will get back into some rotation and power production with this movement, and you can challenge your range of motion during the catch by really trying to twist around as far as possible. This will make the oblique abdominals stretch and contract really hard (that's a good thing).

Preparation

1. Sit on the appropriate-sized stability ball for your height (your legs should be parallel to the floor, with your hips at the same height as your knees). Keep your feet together.

2. Hold a medicine ball over your head, with one hand on each side of the ball.

3. Your partner should be standing 10–15 feet away from you, ready to catch and bounce the ball back.

Movement

4. With a "chopping" motion, throw the ball at the floor, aiming for about halfway between you and your partner. Let go of the ball when your arms are about halfway down, and allow them to continue moving down in a "follow-through" motion. You want the ball to bounce off the floor and into your partner's hands.

5. Your partner will catch the ball and bounce it back to you.

6. Catch the ball with both hands outstretched and bring the ball up into the starting position. Don't stop and hold the ball; use the momentum of the ball to help rotate as far back as you can, and then "spring" back down and bounce the ball. You want to generate as much power and force as you can, which will come from throwing the ball fast.

7. Continue alternating your catch and bounce for a total of 30 repetitions. Complete three sets with about a minute of rest between each one. If you need more of a challenge, you can make this exercise harder by increasing the weight of the medicine ball you are using.

Precautions

Place an exercise mat behind you, in case you fall over backward.

Variations

You can make this exercise more challenging as well. Can you guess how? Lift one foot off the floor.

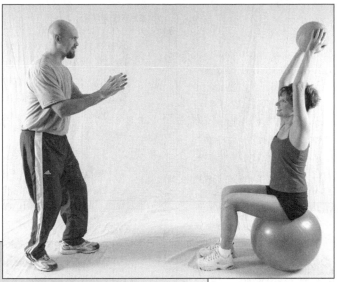

Starting/ending position.

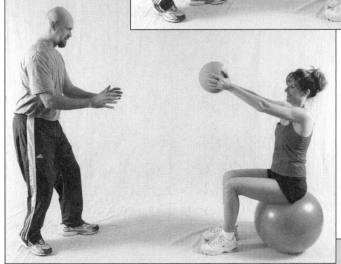

Bounce midpoint.

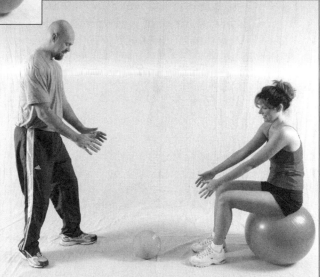

Bounce follow-through.

Balanced Row

Have you ever tried to pull open a door that was too heavy for you? Maybe the wind was pushing it shut, so you had to really pull hard. Remember how your body responded? You probably pulled against the door, but instead of it opening, you pulled yourself closer to the door. This happens because the door was heavier than you, and you didn't have a solid-enough base to pull from. Well, this exercise re-creates that same condition. Why? So you can train your core muscles to stabilize your body while you generate force with your upper body. Next time you go to open a heavy door, it just might fly off its hinges because of your newly found strength.

Preparation

1. Sit on your stability ball with your feet together in front of you.

2. Attach your resistance tubing to your door anchor, or wrap it around a pole at shoulder height (that's shoulder height while you are sitting down). Hold both handles in one hand.

3. Move back from the anchor until all the slack is out of the tubing while your arms are held out in front of you (reaching for the door).

4. Pick up one foot off the floor. It doesn't matter which one; you'll switch in a moment.

Movement

5. Keeping your balance with only one foot on the floor, pull back on the tubing, bringing your elbows to your sides. As you pull back, you will feel the ball try to roll forward. Push on the ground with your foot to counteract this motion and keep yourself in place.

6. When you have the handles as far back as you can, slowly return to the starting point and do another repetition. Do 10–15 repetitions in each set.

7. Switch which foot you are holding up and do another set on this side. Finish two sets on each side.

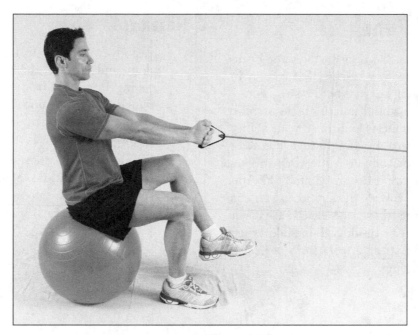

Starting/ending position.

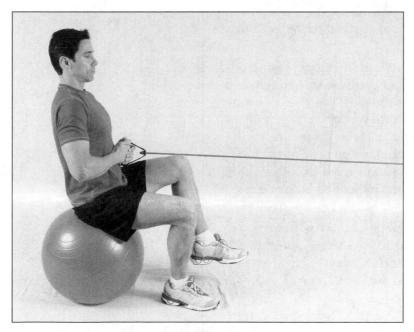

Midpoint position.

Balanced Punch

The balanced punch works on the same principle as the balanced row, except that you try to punch while being resisted by the stretched-out tubing, and without falling off the stability ball. This exercise tests and trains your ability to produce forward-moving power when the ground under you wants to slide away and your body wants to move backward. Sound fun? Your core muscles can control this motion if you contract them correctly, so that's exactly what you are going to do. The results will include a more stable core and a stronger rotation—perfect for when you go surfing.

Preparation

1. Attach your resistance tubing to your door anchor, or wrap it around a pole at about waist level.

2. Sit on your stability ball facing away from the anchor.

3. Hold both ends of the tubing in one hand. Bend your arm so that your hand is next to your shoulder and your elbow is behind you (like you are getting ready to throw a punch). If this is too much resistance, you can hold one end of the tubing in your hand and anchor the other end; you'll build up to holding both ends in time.

4. Scoot the stability ball away from the anchor until all the slack is out of the tubing and it feels like it is just starting to pull you over backward (don't let it).

Movement

5. Lean forward slightly, lift one foot off the floor, and "punch" the hand holding the tubing straight in front of you. As you punch, twist your upper body so that you can press your punch out as far in front of you as possible.

6. Slowly return to the starting position, and do 10–15 repetitions. Switch to the other arm and balancing foot for another set. Do two sets on each side.

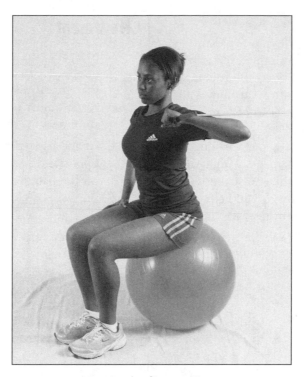

Starting/ending position.

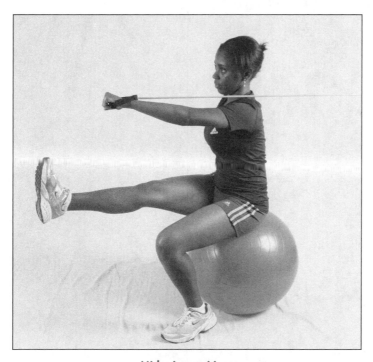

Midpoint position.

Double Circle

The double circle is a fairly simple exercise to do—on the surface. It involves two unstable surfaces that you purposely move around. Why would you do this? To make your core muscles respond to changing stimuli and strengthen their ability to react and keep your torso in place without causing any damage. Although we rarely find ourselves in this unusual position, if you can handle it now, it will help you to manipulate your body in other ways, under other circumstances where it may be needed. It teaches you to move your body in two separate directions at the same time—kind of like patting your belly and rubbing your head at the same time. Sound a little weird? Well, it's not; it's fun and very functional.

Preparation

1. Sit on your stability ball, keeping both feet together and tucked as close to the ball as possible.

2. Hold a medicine ball over your head with both hands.

Movement

3. Start moving the ball over your head in circles. Keep the circles small enough that you aren't moving your lower body to reach out or back—it's all in the arms and shoulders.

4. At the same time, rotate your hips in the opposite direction, making small circles on the ball.

5. Your arms should be moving in one direction and your hips in another. Start slowly and build up speed as you master the movement.

6. Continue these circles for up to 60 seconds; then change directions for another set.

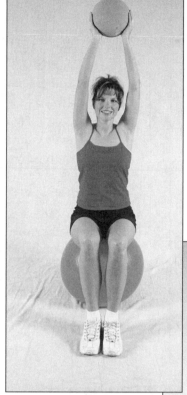

Starting/ending position.

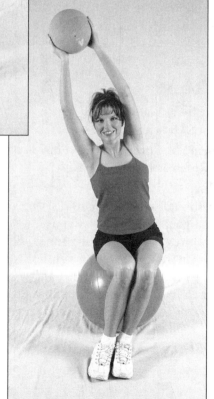

Midpoint through a rotation.

Seated Overhead Catch

You've done some seated throws and bounces, so now I'm going to make it a little more challenging to see if I can get you off balance. The seated overhead catch really stretches the core abdominals and upper-back muscles, and makes the lower-back muscles contract during each catch to offset the momentum of the ball. You need a partner for this exercise, preferably one with good aim because the ball will need to be thrown over your head but within your reach. As your do this exercise, really try to stretch your upper body as high as you can without standing up off the ball. The stretch you feel will actually be the core muscles working to keep you in place and produce power to throw the ball back at your partner (just try not to hurt him or her).

Preparation

1. Sit on your stability ball with your feet together and tucked close to the ball.

2. Hold a medicine ball over your head in both hands. Reach as high as you can while holding the ball.

3. Your partner should stand about 10–15 feet away from you; this is how far you should try to throw the ball, aiming for your partner's chest. You can start with your partner closer until you get the hang of this, and then have him keep stepping back until you can just get the ball to him.

Movement

4. Lean back to about 45 degrees to "wind up" before your throw. Throw the ball to your partner as hard as you can. When you throw the ball, keep your torso as upright and erect as possible.

5. Your partner will catch the ball and throw it back to you. He should aim to throw the ball over your head, just high enough so you can reach it. If you have to lower your arms to catch the ball, your partner threw it too low.

6. Stretch up and catch the ball with your arms straight. Absorb the momentum of the ball quickly before it pulls you over backward.

7. Immediately throw the ball again, using the momentum from the catch as your wind-up. Repeat 10–15 throws for each of three sets.

Precautions

It's a good idea to have a couple of exercise mats behind you, in case you fall over backward.

Variations

Of course, you can make this exercise more of a challenge. Lift one foot off the ground to reduce your stable platform, and then try to keep yourself upright.

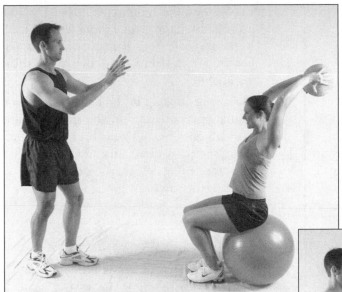

Starting/ending position.

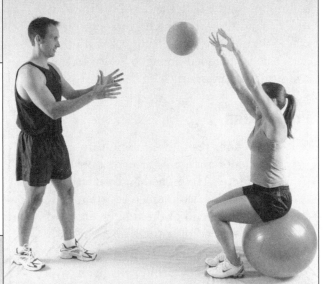

Midpoint throwing position.

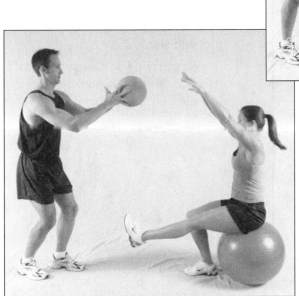

Variation with one foot off the ground.

Bridging Pullover

This exercise combines the elements of stabilization found during ball bridging and the power generation of a resisted sit-up. Together, these two exercises form the bridging pullover, which involves the muscles of the upper and lower back, the abdominals, the shoulder rotators, the hip flexors, and the glutes. That's just about everything, which becomes evident when you do this exercise—meaning you will feel it. Probably the neatest thing about this exercise is that while you are pulling on the tubing and rolling up on the ball, the legs start to work more to aid the core muscles to keep you in place. Because we aren't trying to work the legs, this is an added bonus to your core-conditioning program.

Preparation

1. Loop your resistance tubing through your door anchor or around a pole at waist level. Hold one handle in each hand. If this is too much resistance, anchor one end of the tubing and hold the other end in both hands.

2. Sit on your stability ball, facing away from the anchor. Hold your hands over your head.

3. Lie back on the stability ball, letting it roll up your back until your shoulders are on top of the ball. Your hands should now be pointing back behind you toward the tubing anchor.

4. Hold your hips up in the bridging position so that your knees, hips, and shoulders are in a straight line and your back is straight. Make sure that there isn't any slack in the resistance tubing. If there is, sit up and scoot farther away from the anchor.

Movement

5. Keeping your body in the bridged position, pull the tubing up, over your head, and down until your hands are pointing out in front of you. Keep your arms straight during the entire pull. This will keep the tubing far away from your core, increasing the resistance, and your arms moving in a smooth arc over your body.

6. Slowly return to the starting position, letting the tubing pull you back to where you started. Don't let the tubing snap back quickly—keep your position on the ball nice and stable.

7. As you get good at this exercise, add some speed to your pulls. You can also use a heavier resistance tube to make it harder.

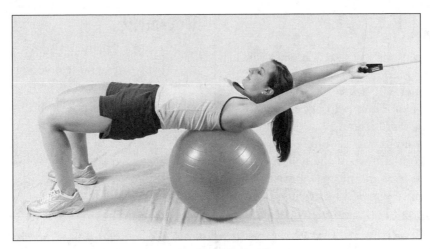

Starting/ending position.

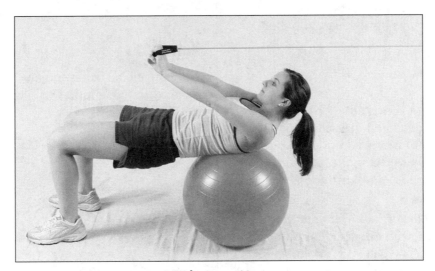

Midpoint position.

Ball Chop

All the other variations of the wood chop positioned you either standing or kneeling. Not this time. Your feet will still be on the ground, but they won't be of much help because you'll be sitting on a ball and leaning over backward. All your feet can do here is provide ballast to help keep you from falling off the ball. Ball chops stretch the core abdominals more than other chops because you will be arching back farther than normal. During the power phase of this movement, the abdominals contract to provide a burst of energy. While all this is happening, the rest of your core muscles, including your upper and lower back, hips, and shoulder rotators, will provide stabilization and, of course, hold the ball.

Preparation

1. Sit on top of your stability ball. Keep your feet together and as close to the ball as you can. If you need to move your feet farther away to feel stable, you can, but work toward keeping them tight against the ball.

2. Hold a medicine ball over your head in both hands, with one hand on each side of the ball. The ball you use should be fairly heavy so that it can generate some momentum when you move it. This momentum is the resistance your muscles will work against to get stronger.

Movement

3. Holding the ball as high as you can, lean back until you feel you are just about to tip over backward.

4. With lots of power, bring the ball forward and down in front of or between your knees.

5. Quickly sit back up, returning the ball back past the starting position to that area where you feel unbalanced, and bring it forward again.

6. Repeat chops until you have done 15–20 in a row. Rest for about 30 seconds and do two more sets.

Variations

If the medicine ball is too much resistance to begin with, use another stability ball until you get the hang of it.

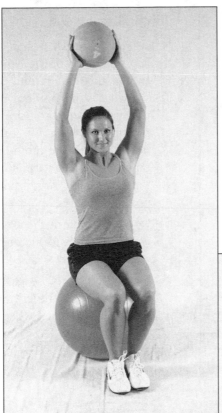

Starting/ending position.

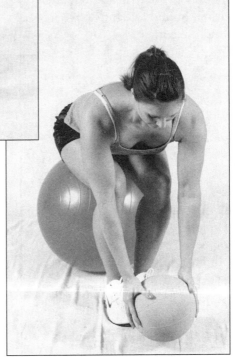

Midpoint position.

Lying Side Pull

This exercise is the first to put you in a position where you can rotate while lying down, and it provides resistance to only one side of your body. The muscles on the side opposite of the hand holding the tubing create the movement, while the side holding the tubing is a stabilizer. This may sound strange because usually whatever side is holding the resistance tubing has to work to move it, but not in this case. We are creating a condition in which the stabilizing force is actually greater than the movement force; it takes more energy to stabilize than to move. All the while, you will be rotating across the top of the ball while in a semibridged position. Sound like fun? Give it a try, and I'll bet you'll like it.

Preparation

1. Attach one end of your resistance tubing to your door anchor or around the bottom of a pole at shoulder level. Hold the other end in one hand. Your other hand rests on your hip.

2. Lie on top of your stability ball so that the arm holding the tubing is reaching out to your side. There can't be any slack in the tubing, so move away from the anchor to get in the right position.

3. Your lower back should be in contact with the stability ball. Your feet should be about a foot apart, to provide some balance. You aren't quite in a bridged position, but you shouldn't let yourself relax over the ball and be loose. Create a little tension in the core by contracting the abdominal muscles just a little bit.

Movement

4. Keep your torso straight as you rotate across the top of the ball away from the tubing anchor. Pretend you are trying to see what is on the floor next to you and that you have to roll over to see it. As you rotate, the arm holding the tubing should be pulling on the tubing to create resistance. Keep your arm straight so the tubing stays as far away from your core as possible.

5. Rotate over until the arm with the tubing is pointing out to the opposite side from where it started.

6. Slowly return to the starting position and complete 10–15 repetitions; then switch sides for another set. Do two sets on each side.

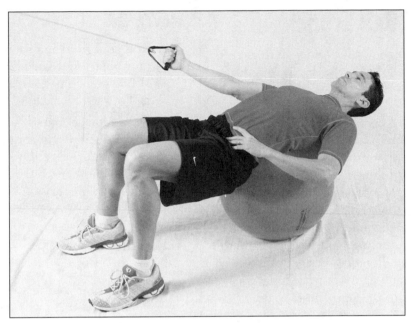

Starting/ending position.

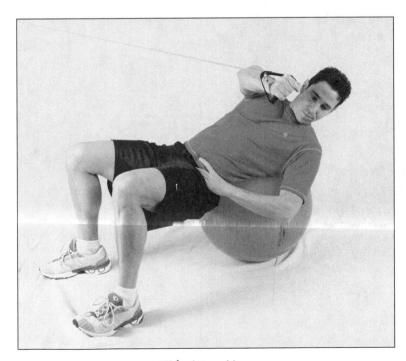

Midpoint position.

Weighted Ball Crunch

Sometimes a crunch just isn't enough to get your abs in shape. Maybe you are looking for an exercise that will make your abs scream at you to stop. Maybe you like that feeling. If you're that kind of person, I've got just the ticket. The weighted ball crunch adds resistance and instability to the good old crunch exercise. And just to make sure that you are really getting enough of a challenge, we are going to do it on only one foot. If you've ever wanted to challenge your abs and really make your core strong, this a great exercise to add to your daily routine. Practice these in private, and then go out and wow your friends at the gym with your skill, strength, and balance.

Preparation

1. Sit on top of your stability ball. Hold a medicine ball with both hands.

2. Lie back on your ball until it rests in your lower back. Arch over the ball so that your head and shoulders are lower than your chest.

3. Hold your medicine ball straight up in the air.

4. Cross one leg over the other so your ankle is resting on your knee.

Movement

5. Roll your head and shoulders up until only your lower back is touching the ball. While you crunch up, push the medicine ball toward the ceiling.

6. Slowly lower yourself back to the starting position and begin another repetition. Complete 20 repetitions; then switch legs and do another set. Two sets on each side should be plenty.

Variations

For more intensity, hold a heavier medicine ball, and/or bring your feet closer to the stability ball. Either of these will amp up the output of your core abdominals.

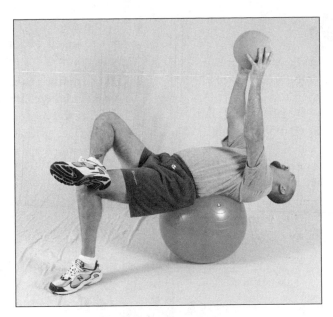

Starting/ending position.

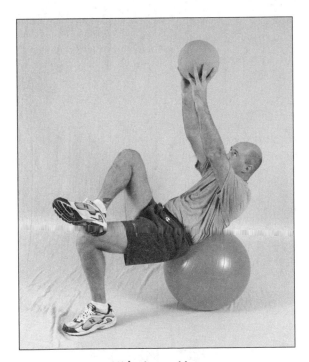

Midpoint position.

Side Touchdown

Are you ready to rotate? Well, you'd better be because that's all you are going to do in this exercise—that and balance on top of the ball again (I just can't stay away from that ball, can you?). The side touchdown challenges your ability to rotate your hips while keeping your feet in one place. This is an exercise that takes some practice and flexibility to complete correctly. If you can't get the full motion right off the bat, go as far as you can, and with practice you'll get there. The flexibility exercises in Chapter 14 will help.

Preparation

1. Lie on your back on your stability ball. Keep your feet out away from the ball and spread apart for balance.

2. Hold another stability ball or your medicine ball over your head with both hands.

Movement

3. Keep your arms straight and rotate to one side, attempting to touch the ball to the floor.

4. When the ball touches the floor, slowly pull yourself back to the starting position and continue on to the other side.

5. Keep rotating back and forth until your set is complete. If you can't touch the floor in the beginning, really push yourself with each repetition. I'll bet you'll get closer and closer.

Precautions

With the amount of rotation involved in this exercise, if you feel any pain or muscle spasms in your lower back, discontinue this exercise and consult with your doctor.

Variations

If you are nowhere near touching the floor, use a stability ball instead of a medicine ball. Work your way to using the medicine ball over time as your core gets stronger.

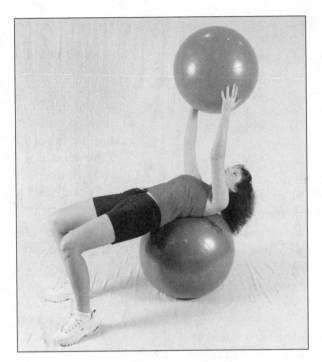

Starting/ending position.

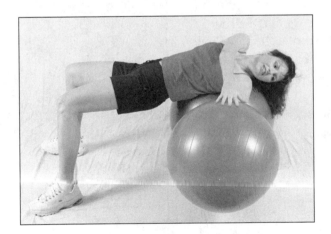

Midpoint position.

Two-Ball Stabilizer

I've saved the best for last. This exercise challenges not only your core muscles, but just about every muscle in your body. It's not really an arm or leg exercise because, without the core providing the bulk of the stabilization, you wouldn't even get off the ground. When you are off the ground, your core is what keeps you there. This exercise will definitely tighten up every muscle you can think of and may introduce you to muscles you didn't know existed. Two-ball stabilizers will put that finishing touch on an already-strong core, plus give you ninja-like balance and agility.

Preparation

1. You need two stability balls and either an exercise mat or a carpeted surface for this exercise. The balls don't have to be the same size.

2. Kneel in front of one stability ball, and place your hands just to each side of the top of the ball.

3. Bend your knees and place your feet on top of the other ball. At this point, only your knees are still touching the floor; your hands and feet are both on stability balls.

Movement

4. In one smooth motion, push up with your hands and out with your feet until your entire body is off the floor and supported on the stability balls. You may be in a piked position to start. Work toward bringing your hips down so that your shoulders, hips, knees, and feet are all in a straight line. This should look like you are doing push-ups on top of stability balls.

5. Hold this position for up to 60 seconds, and then slowly relax back to the floor. Rest for 15–20 seconds before your next set.

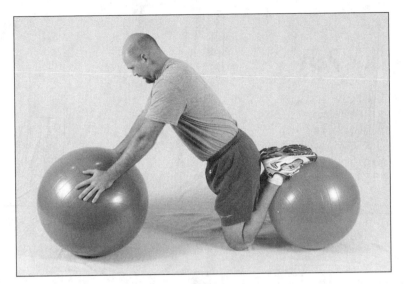

Starting/ending position.

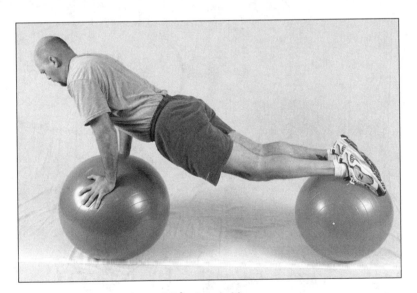

Midpoint position.

In This Part

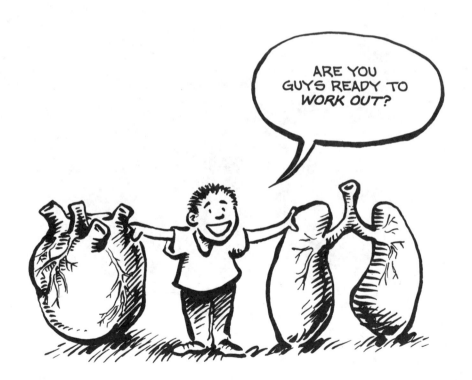

Part 3

Keeping in Touch

A well-rounded core-conditioning program isn't all about the isolated exercises you do. A complete program includes proper cardiovascular training for that big heart muscle right in the middle of your core, and a healthy dose of flexibility training to keep you limber and ready for more. This final part provides all the details you need to finish up your core-conditioning program in style. To end it all, the final chapter gives you some helpful hints on keeping your motivation level high and how to track your workouts for future success.

In This Chapter

- ◆ Using cardiovascular exercise to strengthen the core
- ◆ What's a core cardio exercise and what's not
- ◆ How much, how often, and how to
- ◆ Determining your target heart rate

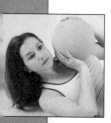 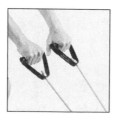 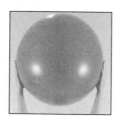 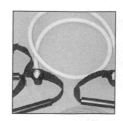 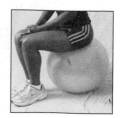 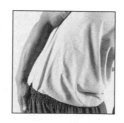

Core Cardio

A truly fit person's core has both muscular strength and muscular endurance. However, we have yet to explore the most important muscle in your core. This is a muscle you use even when you aren't moving. This muscle has to be kept in shape because it keeps you alive. It's your heart, a big piece of muscle that is constantly working and is technically part of your core. Without your heart, the other core muscles couldn't do their jobs because the heart supplies other muscles with blood, oxygen, and nutrients.

The central theme of your core-conditioning workout comes from the strengthening exercises of the previous nine chapters, but to get the full effect of working the core, you have to include a good dose of cardiovascular exercise. This chapter explores the different types of cardiovascular exercise that work your heart and core muscles at the same time, giving you the total workout your body deserves.

Multidirectional Cardio

As you've learned from the other exercises in this book, the core muscles don't just move in one direction, but they incorporate bending, twisting, pushing, and pulling all at once. To train the core, you have to move in as many directions as you can at one time. If you look at many typical cardiovascular workouts, you'll find that only a small part of the core is engaged, while the muscles in the arms or legs do most of the work. We need to find cardio exercises that engage the torso to provide rotation and stability while the arms and legs assist in providing movement.

Unfortunately, the most popular cardio exercises don't do this. For instance, running on a treadmill barely engages the core at all—the legs do all the work. Riding a stationary bike is even worse because the core is stabilized by the seat and doesn't have to work. Elliptical trainers and stair-climbers don't help, either—again, the legs are working while you hold on to a bar and keep your torso still. We have to make the core muscles work by having them actually do something.

Don't Throw It Out _____

A core cardio workout includes exercises that make the core muscles work to either provide movement or stability. Treadmills, stationary bikes, elliptical trainers, and stair-climbers don't meet this criteria.

Getting Off the Treadmill

Without treadmills, stair-climbers, stationary bikes, or elliptical trainers, most people wouldn't know what to do for their cardiovascular workouts. Because you want to involve your core muscles as well as get your heart rate up, we have to go beyond the most popular machines and find a few that really help us meet our goals. Only five types of cardiovascular exercises can do this: rowing machines, cross-country skiing, swimming, skating, and smooth-water kayaking. As a bonus, each of these exercises is a whole lot cheaper than buying a treadmill, and a lot more fun because you get to go outside and play.

Rowing Machines

I believe rowing machines are one of the most overlooked exercise methods out there today. Did you know that people actually compete in rowing machine "races" all over the world? It's true! Rowing machines measure the distance you have "rowed," so a race distance is determined and whoever gets there first wins. It's really quite fun to watch.

What makes rowing machines such a good core workout is that they make you move your arms and your legs, with your torso tying it all together. Your core muscles have to contract to stabilize your body while you row; otherwise, you wouldn't be able to pull on the handle. The key to getting the most core work from a rowing-machine workout is to make sure you are sitting up straight the entire time. Your entire abdominal area, lower back, upper back, and shoulders are working to keep your body stabilized and your spine good and straight while your legs push and your arms pull—it's got just about everything.

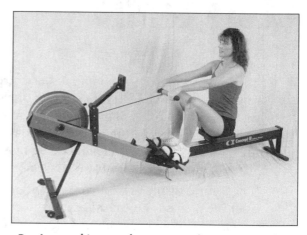

Rowing machines work your arms, legs, core muscles, and heart all at the same time.

Cross-Country Skiing

No snow? No problem. Cross-country skiing can be done outside if there's snow or inside on a machine. Studies have shown that you burn more calories during a cross-country skiing workout than any other type of exercise you can think of. I won't kid you—it's not easy, but it's worth it. Unlike treadmills, ellipticals, or stair-climbers, cross-country skiing makes you use your arms and legs together in a standing position. Your arms actually help propel your body instead of just moving in space or holding on to a handrail. If you do this outside, the arms push poles into the snow; inside, the arms pull on handles attached to cables. Either way, your arms have to exert force to move, and your core muscles must help the upper body rotate during this movement.

Cross-country skiing machines were very popular in the 1980s but have almost dropped off the fitness scene. I think the major contributor to their demise was their difficulty. This isn't an exercise that you can just jump on and be good at—it takes practice. Most people weren't willing to put in the practice to get the results (they weren't nearly as dedicated as you are). Those who did stick with it ended up with incredible fitness levels and core muscles to be envious of.

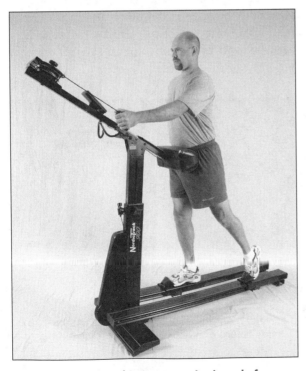

The NordicTrack is the most popular brand of cross-country skiing machine made and really works all the core muscles at one time.

Swimming

Want a fun workout where you don't sweat? Get in the pool. Swimming has long been an excellent form of cardiovascular exercise. When I look at the bodies of the best swimmers, I see solid core muscles. These people are totally in shape and usually don't have an ounce of fat on them. I think they may be on to something.

Swimming is a great cardiovascular workout, but it also relies on the core muscles to get it done. Swimming is not just about how fast you can kick your feet or move your arms; it's really about how well you can rotate your body—especially your torso. Professional swimmers will tell you that the more time you can spend on your side in the water, the faster you will be. The only way to move from side to side is to rotate your torso. When you rotate your torso, your arms and legs move more efficiently, making you a better swimmer. So with every stroke, your entire body, including your core, is getting a workout.

Suck It In

When swimming laps at your local pool or lake, concentrate on rotating your body from side to side to engage all your core muscles and keep your heart rate up the entire workout.

Roller and Ice Skating

How long has it been since you've laced up a pair of roller or ice skates? Since you were a kid? Kids love to skate because it's fun. I don't think it gets any less fun as you get older; we just starting thinking of it as more of an exercise than a fun activity. That's a bad way to think about skating—it's still fun! With the invention of inline skating, this form of exercise has seen an elevation from a kid's activity to a legitimate form of adult exercise.

Skating is a good core-conditioning and cardio workout because you can't skate well without moving your arms and rotating your body from side to side. The core muscles provide all this rotation and a stable base for your legs to push from. You won't really feel the core muscles working that much during skating, but that's just because the alternating contractions from side to side give each muscle a little rest between movements. Skating is a great reason to get outside to exercise, can be done at skating rinks during bad weather, and is always a fun family activity.

Don't Throw It Out

If you go skating, remember to wear knee pads, elbow pads, gloves, and a protective helmet. Skating can be a fun exercise, but it also needs to be safe.

Kayaking

When you think of kayaking, are you imagining a guy stuffed into a little boat splashing through the rapids on some out-of-control river? Well, that's not the type of kayaking I have in mind for you. I'm talking about smooth-water kayaking, the kind done on lakes, on slow-moving rivers, and along the shores of the ocean. No big rocks or waterfalls for us. Pulling yourself out of the water after getting tossed around is not the kind of workout I normally recommend.

Smooth-water kayaking is a great workout that's also a little different from anything else out there. The biggest challenge is that all the work is done by your core and your arms; your legs don't do anything. Upper-body cardiovascular workouts have long been known for making your heart stronger. The issue most people have with it is how hard it is. It's hard only because you haven't gotten used to it! Once you give kayaking a try, you'll probably fall in love with it. Your heart gets a workout, your core gets to provide all the rotation (which it loves to do), and you get to have some fun.

Kayaking for your core cardio workout changes things up quite a bit. No longer can the large muscles in your legs help you out. Your torso and your arms have to provide all the propulsion to move you through the water. That's a big chore, but there are plenty of muscles to get it done. When you paddle a kayak correctly, the arms really don't do much more than hold on to the paddle. The core muscles provide most of the movement—and, therefore, get most of the results.

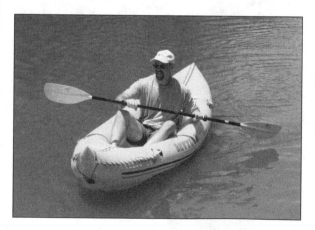

Kayaking on slow-moving water is a great way to enjoy nature and get your core cardio workout at the same time.

How Much and How Often

Hopefully you haven't been brainwashed into believing that you have to do an hour of cardiovascular work every day to make any difference. That old belief has no scientific basis whatsoever, so forget everything you have ever heard about how hard it is to get your cardio workout done. Just like the other core-conditioning exercises, a little goes a long way. Now, I can't say that only 5–10 minutes a day is enough for everybody, but it might be enough for you if you haven't been doing anything so far. The key to finding the right amount of cardiovascular work is just like deciding how much core conditioning to do: just a little bit more than you are used to doing.

A good goal for your cardiovascular workout is 30 minutes every day, but you can split that up just like you can split up your core-conditioning workout. Three 10-minute sessions is the same as 30 straight minutes. If you want, you can do a little more on some days and a little less on other days. I know you all have different life schedules and that sometimes getting 30 minutes of cardio into your day is impossible. If you can't get it one day, fine, make up for it later—that's called *exercise accumulation*. When I have to skip a day for some reason, such as when I have a bad headache, I spread that workout over the next three days and do 40 minutes each day to make up for it. See how simple that is?

Getting Defined

Exercise accumulation is the result of adding up smaller exercise sessions until you reach the total time you set as your goal. Over a week, 20 minutes each day of core conditioning and core cardio equals a total of more than 4½ hours of exercise!

Targeting Your Heart Rate

The question I get asked the most concerning cardiovascular exercise is "How hard do I have to work?" That's a great question. Too often I see people "getting their cardio workout" when all they are really doing is casually strolling around the block. Just like any other type of workout, your body will respond to it and improve only if it has to. Remember that our bodies are really lazy—they don't improve unless we make them improve. When it comes to cardio workouts, the best way to gauge your intensity and actually make progress is to monitor your heart rate.

Your target heart rate for cardio exercise is based on your age and your resting heart rate. There is a maximum speed that your heart can beat, appropriately called your maximum heart rate (those scientist guys really make things technical). You can make a pretty good estimation of your maximum heart rate by subtracting your age from 220. For example, if you are 30 years old, your estimated maximum heart rate is 190 beats a minute (pretty fast).

The next thing you have to do is find out what your resting heart rate is. To do this, sit quietly for about 5 minutes, and then find your pulse in your neck or wrist, and count how many beats you feel in 1 minute. That's your resting heart rate.

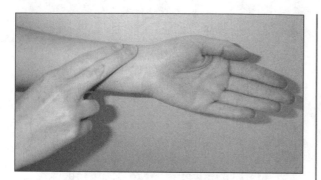

Use your index and middle fingers to find your pulse at your wrist. Your pulse point is in the groove just below your palm on the thumb side.

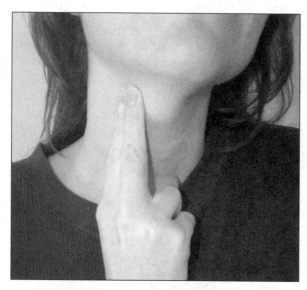

Use your index and middle fingers to find your pulse on the side of your neck. Your pulse point is in the groove just to either side of the center of your neck.

Our final step is a little more complicated and involves some math that is best left to a calculator (unless you can multiply fractions in your head). Subtract your resting heart rate from your maximum heart rate. Now multiply that number by 0.6 and 0.8 (you will have two numbers). Finally, add your resting heart rate to each of these numbers. This is your target heart rate range. Here's an example:

1. Subtract your age from 220. (220 – 30 = 190)
2. Subtract your resting heart rate from 190. (190 – 70 = 120)
3. Multiply 120 by 0.6 and 0.8. (120 × 0.6 = 72, 120 × 0.8 = 96)
4. Add your resting heart rate to each number. (72 + 70 = 142, 96 + 70 = 166)
5. Your target heart rate is between 142 and 166.

With your target heart rate range calculated, all you have to do now is make sure that your heart rate is within this range while you work out. Stop every 10–15 minutes and check your pulse. It's hard to count that many beats in a minute because your heart will be beating really fast, so just count for 15 seconds and multiply by 4. As long as you are within your range and you feel like you are working, keep going. It is possible to be in your heart rate range and not be working hard enough, so every now and then, push yourself a little faster or harder.

The Least You Need to Know

◆ Core cardio exercises have to involve your core muscles as part of the movement. Treadmills, stationary bikes, elliptical trainers, and stair-climbers don't cut it.

◆ The best exercises for core cardio are rowing machines, cross-country skiing, swimming, skating, and kayaking.

◆ Shoot for a total of 30 minutes of cardio work every day. If you can't get it all in on one day, make up for it later.

◆ Calculate your target heart rate range to make sure you are working as hard as you need to, but not too hard.

In This Chapter

- Why it's important to stretch after a workout

- The best time to stretch

- Cooling down after a workout

- Twisting, tucking, leaning, and rolling: a dozen great stretches

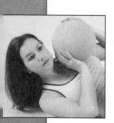
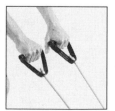
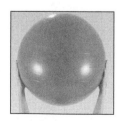
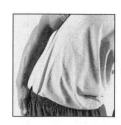
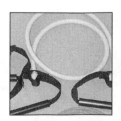
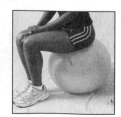

Chapter 14

Stretch It Out

I once met a guy named Larry who complained that his muscles ached and sometimes cramped after his workouts. Larry had been following a great exercise program, but he was skipping the last part of it because he didn't think it was helping him meet his goals. Larry wasn't stretching.

When you walk away from a workout, you should feel relaxed, energized, and ready to move on to the next part of your day. If you finish your workout with a strenuous exercise that has left you tired and sweaty, with your muscles all tensed up, I doubt you are in a happy place. Every time you work a muscle, you need to rest it. After a muscle has been contracted, it needs to be stretched—it's that simple. This chapter teaches you how to finish your workouts with relaxing stretches that will leave you feeling good about your workout.

Why Should You Stretch?

You eat and sleep because you have to. You exercise because you need to (and because you like it). You should stretch because it's good for you (just like your mother used to say). For as long as I can remember, exercise professionals have recommended flexibility training as an essential part of an exercise program. They didn't suggest that you do some stretching only if you felt like it or only if you had time. Stretching is just as important as core-conditioning exercises and cardiovascular exercises—but in a different way.

I've known a lot of people who were absolutely diligent in getting their daily exercise but would spend less than a minute stretching—and even then, they were just going through the motions. When a muscle contracts and produces force, a lot of things happen inside the body. For instance, lactic acid is formed and builds up in the muscle. When enough lactic acid is produced, the muscle stops working and you get tired. If you stop exercising, the lactic acid slowly leaves the muscles—but what if there were a way to speed up that process? There is: stretching (but you guessed that one).

Aside from some chemical advantages, stretching a tired muscle can help it recover from the exercise faster. This gets you back to working out again even faster (yea!). It's also been said that being more flexible can help you move more easily and feel better all day long. We don't want muscles to cramp or joints to feel tight. If you could move all day long and your body always felt loose and relaxed, wouldn't that be worth a few extra minutes of your time? I believe it would. If you are still skeptical, just try it for a few days; I guarantee you will convert to a stretching fanatic.

> **Six-Pack Says**
>
> Flexibility, strength, and cardiovascular endurance are all equally important parts of the fitness equation. Leave one part out, and your program won't give you all the results you expect.
>
> —Chat Williams, personal trainer

Timing Is Everything

The debate over when is the best time to stretch has been going on in the fitness community for a long time. There are basically two trains of thought: 1) stretch after you have finished all your exercises, and 2) stretch each muscle immediately after you use it. Both sides have some compelling positives and negatives, and both agree that stretching should always be done after a muscle has been worked, never before. The important point is that a warm muscle will stretch easier than a cold one because a warm muscle has a higher core temperature and more localized blood flow. So it doesn't really matter whether you wait until the end of your entire workout or stretch after each exercise, as long as you never stretch before your workout.

Cooling down after a workout is always a good idea. By cooling down, I don't mean standing in front of the air-conditioner. Cooling down refers to a time when your heart rate returns to normal, you stop sweating, and you feel relaxed. Because stretching doesn't take much effort or movement, it fits the bill nicely. Use stretching as your cool-down time, and you will have accomplished two things at once. To focus on your stretching and also get your cool-down time in, find a quiet place where you have plenty of room to lie down and relax. This is also a good time to drink some water and towel off, if you're sweaty.

Besides not stretching, the second problem I see a lot is that people don't stretch long enough. To increase your flexibility and get all the benefits of a stretch, you need to hold each stretch for 30 to 60 seconds. Most of us can't sit still for a solid minute, let alone hold a stretch that long; that's why you have a range of time with an ultimate goal at the end. If you can stretch for only 30 seconds, I'll take it. As you practice, you'll get better and will be able to stretch for longer.

I've included the top 12 stretches for the core in this chapter. If you did every one of them, your stretching time would be less than 30 minutes, but you don't have to do all of them every day. You should pick the stretches that feel the best to you and that give you the most relaxed feeling afterward. Try each stretch and work on the ones that seem challenging at first; those are the areas where you need the most improvement in flexibility.

> **Don't Throw It Out**
>
> Hold each stretch at the point you just start to feel the strain. A stretch shouldn't hurt, so if you feel pain, back off a little.

Inverted Superman

You will feel this stretch through the abdominals (from your pelvis to your ribs), across your chest, and under your arms. It's a lot like the stretch you do when you first wake up, but you can't go back to sleep right now.

Targets

- ◆ Abdominals
- ◆ Hip flexors
- ◆ Shoulders
- ◆ Chest

Directions

1. Lie down on your back on a carpeted surface or an exercise mat.

2. Point your toes away from you, and reach out over your head with both arms.

3. Try to make your body as long as you can, pushing your toes away from you and your hands out over your head.

4. It's okay to arch your back a little to get the biggest stretch possible. Your goal is to get to the point that you can lay your arms flat on the floor over your head (all the way from your shoulders to your hands).

5. Take deep breaths while you hold this position for up to 60 seconds, but keep trying to reach a little farther. Rest for a few seconds and repeat twice more.

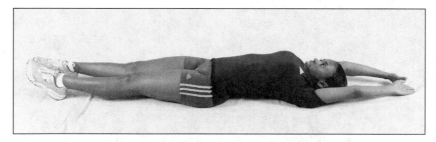

Inverted Superman stretch—make yourself as long as you can.

Standing Side Reach

The effects of this stretch will be felt mainly down your side, from just under your shoulder to your lower ribs, and across the outside of your hips.

Targets

- ◆ Abdominals
- ◆ Chest
- ◆ Shoulders
- ◆ Lower back
- ◆ Hip flexors
- ◆ Hip extensors

Directions

1. Stand with your feet slightly wider than shoulder-width apart. Keep your hands down at your sides.

2. Reach one hand up over your head as high as you can, while the other hand stays against your leg.

3. Slowly lean over to one side, sliding your hand down your leg as far as possible. The hand in the air reaches out and over your head as far as possible (don't bend your elbow).

4. Breathe deeply and hold this position for up to 60 seconds while you keep trying to reach a little further.

5. Relax and rest for a moment, then repeat on the other side. Complete two stretches on each side.

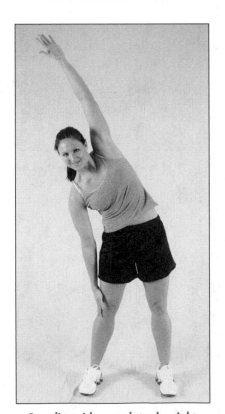

Standing side stretch to the left.　　　Standing side stretch to the right.

Seated Pretzel

You'll feel this stretch in your lower back and middle back, through the hip that is bent, and diagonally across your abdominals.

Targets

- ◆ Lower back
- ◆ Upper back
- ◆ Oblique abdominals
- ◆ Hip flexors
- ◆ Hip extensors

Directions

1. Sit on the floor on a carpeted surface or an exercise mat. Place your legs straight out in front of you.

2. Bend one leg up and cross it over the other leg so that your foot is on the floor next to the other knee.

3. If you crossed your left knee over your right leg (see the left photo below), place your right elbow on the outside of the left knee (the bent knee). Your other hand is on the floor behind you supporting your upper body.

4. Breathe deeply and push against your knee to help twist your upper body to the right as far as possible. Do not let your hips leave the floor.

5. Hold this position for up to 60 seconds; keep breathing.

6. Relax for a moment and repeat on the other side. Cross your right leg over your left leg, place your left elbow on your right knee, and twist.

7. Repeat the stretch for each side twice.

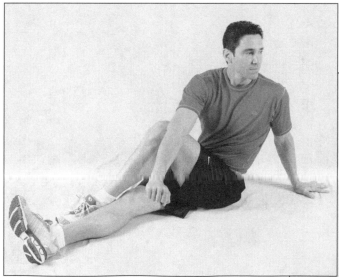

Seated pretzel stretch to the left.

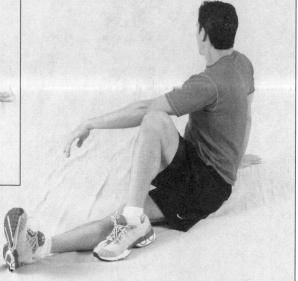

Seated pretzel stretch to the right.

Twisted Cross

This stretch will be felt mainly in your lower back, a little in your middle and upper back, and through your hips, possibly out to your knees.

Targets

- ◆ Oblique abdominals
- ◆ Lower back
- ◆ Hip extensors

Directions

1. Lie on the floor on your back on a carpeted surface or an exercise mat.
2. Bend your knees and slide your feet up until they are about a foot away from your butt.

3. Lay your arms out to your sides, palms up and relaxed.
4. Breathe deeply as you roll your knees over to one side. As you let them fall toward the floor, keep your feet together. This means one foot will leave the floor and rest on the bottom foot.
5. Press your knees toward the floor as far as you can. The goal is to lay your knees on the floor. Be sure to keep your shoulders down. If your upper body starts to roll over, stop and relax into the stretch right there.
6. Hold this position for up to 60 seconds. Keep trying to push your knees down for more stretch.
7. Relax, bring your knees back up to the starting position, and roll to the other side for another stretch. Stretch each side twice.

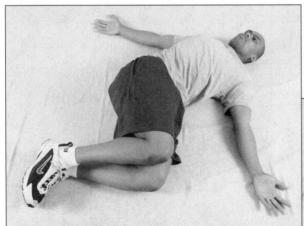

Twisted cross stretch to the left side.

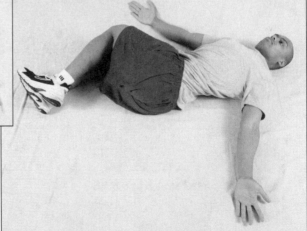

Twisted cross stretch to the right side.

Diagonal Hips

You will feel this stretch deep inside the hip that is pulled, across your butt, and into your lower back.

Targets

- Lower back
- Hip extensors

Directions

1. Lie on your back using either an exercise mat or a carpeted surface.
2. Keep your legs together and your arms down at your sides.

3. Bring your right knee up toward your chest, and grab hold of that knee with your left hand.
4. You have to really let your leg relax now. Your left hand will hold your leg up. Relax your hips and leg, and let your foot drop so it hangs in the air.
5. Keeping your shoulders and hips on the floor, pull your knee across your body toward your left shoulder. If you aren't feeling the stretch, your leg isn't relaxed enough—there are muscles still tightened up. Let it all go!
6. Hold the stretch for up to 60 seconds; then relax that leg and repeat on the other side by pulling the left leg across the body with your right hand. Repeat each leg twice.

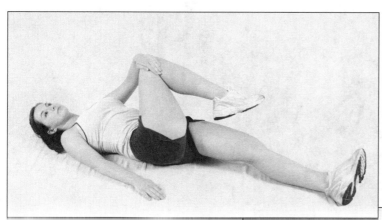

Diagonal hips stretch for the right leg.

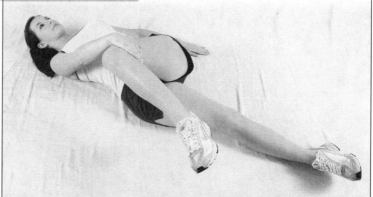

Diagonal hips stretch for the left leg.

Tuck

The effects of this stretch will mostly be on your lower back, but depending on how tight you are, you may feel it up into your middle and upper back, and across your butt.

Targets

- ◆ Lower back
- ◆ Hip extensors
- ◆ Middle back

Directions

1. Lie on your back on an exercise mat or a carpeted surface.

2. Reach under your knees with both hands and pull your knees in toward your chest.

3. Tuck your chin to your chest and lift your shoulders and head off the floor.

4. Try to make yourself into as small a ball as possible; then hold the stretch for up to 60 seconds.

5. Relax for a few moments and repeat two more times.

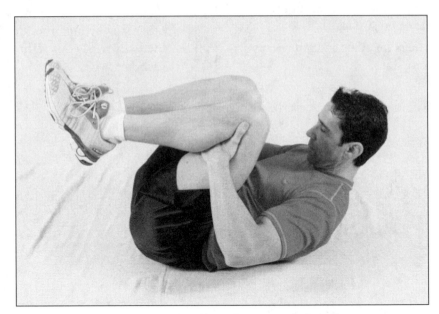

The tuck stretch is like rolling into a little ball.

Ball Arc

This stretch is probably the most intense stretch you can do for the abdominals and chest. It's the only stretch in this chapter that requires the use of a piece of equipment: a stability ball. If you have any back problems, skip this stretch because it will put your body into extreme hyper-extension and could aggravate an injured back.

Targets

◆ Abdominals
◆ Hip flexors
◆ Chest
◆ Shoulders

Directions

1. Lie across the top of your stability ball so that the ball is in the middle of your back.

2. Stretch your legs away from you as far as possible, keeping your heels on the floor and pointing your toes.

3. Reach over your head with both arms.

4. Let your back muscles relax and stretch over the top of the ball. Try to reach back and down with your arms until you can touch the floor.

5. Your head and neck should be relaxed and will probably be lower than your chest, so keep breathing deeply throughout the stretch.

6. Hold this position for up to 60 seconds, sit back up on the ball, relax for a few moments, and then repeat two more times.

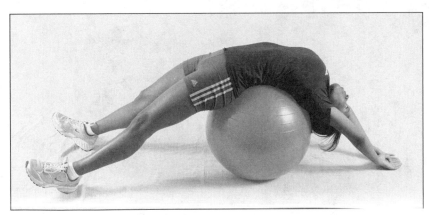

Ball arc stretch using a stability ball.

Leaning Tower

You'll feel this stretch all the way down your spine and into your hips. If you feel a stretch in your hamstrings, it just means your hips are really tight.

Targets

◆ Hip extensors
◆ Lower back
◆ Middle back
◆ Upper back

Directions

1. Stand with your feet together with a little bit of bend in your knees (don't keep them locked).

2. Bend forward and wrap your arms around your legs just above your knees. Try to grab hold of your wrists instead of interlocking your fingers.

3. Let your head and neck relax, but keep taking deep breaths to keep from getting lightheaded.

4. Using your arms to pull, bring your chest down as close to your knees as you can.

5. Hold this position for up to 60 seconds. Stand back up and relax for a few moments; then repeat two more times.

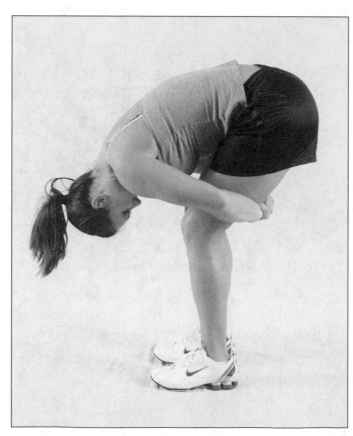

Leaning tower stretch for the back and hips.

Twist and Hold

This stretch actually gets all the little muscles up and down your spine, but you can't really feel them because the larger surface muscles have more nerve endings. You'll feel the twisting of all the muscles up and down your back, and into your hips a little bit.

Targets

◆ Lower back

◆ Oblique abdominals

◆ Hip extensors

◆ Middle back

Directions

1. Stand with your feet shoulder-width apart.

2. Either interlock your fingers or grasp each arm at the wrist. Hold your hands in front of you about chest level, elbows out to the sides.

3. Keep your feet in place, allow your knees to bend a little bit, and rotate your entire body like you are trying to look behind you.

4. When you have twisted as far as you can, hold this position for up to 60 seconds. Keep trying to rotate a little farther all the time.

5. Relax and twist in the other direction. Alternate left and right twists twice on each side.

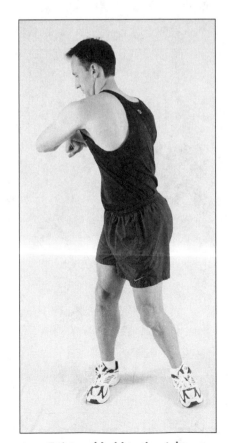

Twist and hold to the left.   Twist and hold to the right.

Bend and Twist

This stretch really gets at only a couple of muscle groups, but it does so in a big way. You'll feel this in your lower back, across your butt, and possibly down your hamstrings, if your hips are really tight.

Targets

- ◆ Hip extensors
- ◆ Lower back

Directions

1. Stand with your feet slightly wider than shoulder-width apart.

2. Bend at the waist as far as you can while keeping your back straight. Let your arms hang down in front of you.

3. When you have bent over as far as you can, twist your body so that your hands are reaching for the toes on one foot. This puts a bit of rotation into your stretch.

4. Keep your back as straight as possible. If you can't reach your toes yet, that's okay; just stretch as far as you can right now.

5. Hold this stretch for up to 60 seconds. Keep taking deep breaths so you don't get lightheaded.

6. Stand back up, relax for a few seconds, and repeat the stretch toward the other foot. Repeat each side two times.

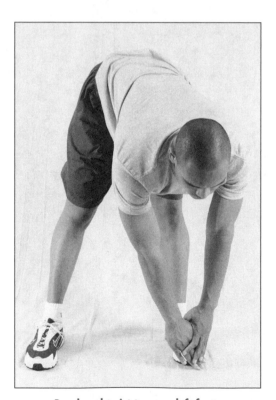

Bend and twist to your left foot.

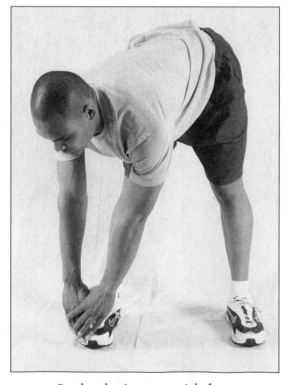

Bend and twist to your right foot.

Over-Roll

When you do this stretch, you may feel some pressure on your upper back, shoulders, and neck, but that's just the weight of your body pushing into the floor. The actual stretch is taking place in your lower back and hips.

Targets

◆ Middle back
◆ Lower back
◆ Hip extensors

Directions

1. Lie on your back on a carpeted surface or an exercise mat.

2. Lay your arms out to your sides, palms down. Keep your feet together and legs straight.

3. Using your arms and hands to push against the floor and assist your movement, slowly lift your legs up and over your body until your lower back comes up off the floor.

4. Once your feet move past your head, or your lower back comes off the floor, relax your legs and attempt to bring your knees toward your chest as much as possible (but don't bend your knees).

5. Hold this position for up to 60 seconds.

6. If your middle back comes off the floor, you've gone too far. You may not feel much of a stretch in your lower back and hips, but it's there.

7. Let your feet back down to the floor, relax a few moments, and repeat this stretch two more times.

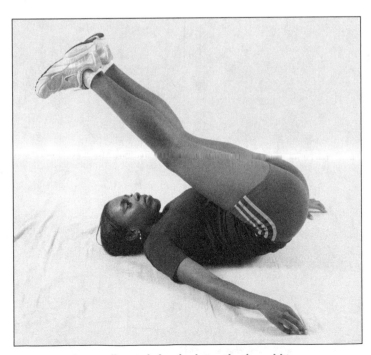

Over-roll stretch for the lower back and hips.

Cat

This last stretch is something I see my cats doing all the time. They've got the right idea because you will feel this on both sides of your spine: the lower back and the abdominals.

Targets

- ◆ Lower back
- ◆ Middle back
- ◆ Abdominals
- ◆ Chest

Directions

1. Kneel on the floor on your hands and knees. Place your hands directly under your shoulders, and your knees directly under your hips.

2. Keep your knees together, your hands shoulder-width apart.

3. Begin by letting your core drop toward the floor, kind of like an old, sagging horse. Really push your abdominals toward the floor.

4. Hold this position for about 30 seconds.

5. Now lift your back in the air as far as you can. Pretend your spine is attached to a string that is being pulled up. Arch your back all the way from your shoulders to your hips.

6. Hold this position for about 30 seconds.

7. Alternate down and up positions until you have finished three stretches of each.

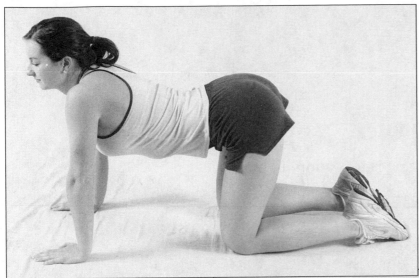

Down position for cat stretch.

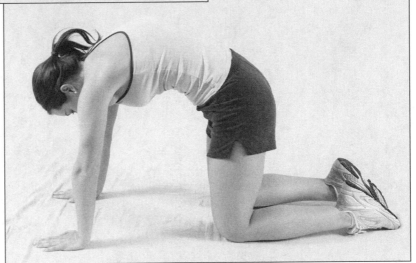

Up position for cat stretch.

In This Chapter

- ◆ Keeping your motivation high
- ◆ Measuring your progress
- ◆ Training with a pro
- ◆ Being at your best

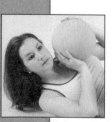
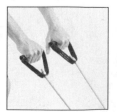
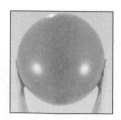
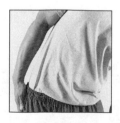
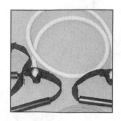
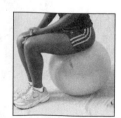

Chapter 15

Staying on Track

The hardest part of a core-conditioning program is not being able to see the results in the mirror. With a body-sculpting or weight-training program, those large surface muscles make dramatic changes that you can visually see. You have to remember that core conditioning is about training the muscles deeper inside the body that help keep you lined up and in good shape. This type of training builds a solid foundation for body sculpting or weight training. Like the foundation of your house, you probably can't see a lot of it, but you know it's working if your house doesn't fall down. It's the same way with core conditioning: you will know it's working because you feel it working. You kind of have to learn to "see" with your brain and feel how your body is changing, visualizing that in your mind.

The motivation to keep with a core-conditioning program has to come from within. This is not about looking better, but actually being better. A book cannot be judged by its cover, and neither can your body. It's what's happening inside that makes the biggest difference—and that's where core conditioning has the strongest effect.

Staying on Schedule

I believe the best way to track your progress and move your program forward is to keep a journal. This doesn't have to be anything fancy or special—just a plain old notebook where you can write down your daily workout (see Appendix C for an example). Journaling is just like keeping a diary of your workouts. Include the exercises you do, the number of reps and sets and time, plus how you feel about each workout. Keeping track of each exercise gives you a history to look back on and see how far you have come. If you want motivation, look back at a journal from several weeks or months ago and compare that to what you are doing now. If you have been pushing yourself a little bit each day, you will be able to see the progress right there on paper. That's solid proof you are on track and moving ahead.

> ### Six-Pack Says
>
> Even the most enthusiastic person will falter if they don't remember why they started training in the first place. Learning to embrace how your body changes without visual results is the characteristic of a motivated and successful person.
>
> —Edwin Cole, fitness enthusiast and motivational speaker

Journaling can also be a good source of motivation to help you get back on schedule if you get too busy and your workouts fall by the wayside. Far too often clients do great and then have to stop working out for some reason. When they come back in again, they are worried that they'll have to start all over and that they've lost all the progress they made. To alleviate their worries, I tell them (and I'm telling you) that very rarely will your body revert to its "pre-training" state. You will always retain some of that progress, even if it's just the knowledge of how to do the exercises correctly. Knowledge is power and is usually the biggest obstacle a person has to overcome when starting a new exercise program.

If you've fallen off the wagon for a while, don't worry. Those movement patterns you learned long ago are still stored in your brain. Now you just have to get out your journal and jump back into your routine. You'll quickly find yourself getting back to your old success levels even faster than the first time around. Having a record of how you progressed in the first place will keep you aware of what you are capable of. If you did it once, you can do it again (and better this time)!

Working with a Personal Trainer

I suggest that you meet with a professional personal trainer from time to time to give your program a boost. Even I, as a personal trainer, use other trainers and coaches to give me a kick in the pants from time to time and push me to new levels. A personal trainer can help you measure your progress, assist you in evaluating whether you are doing exercises correctly, and provide you with another means of motivation. I always want to give my trainer or coach a positive report when I see him. It pushes me to reach new goals and keep working harder.

You don't have to work with a trainer all the time. Once every few weeks, or even once a month for a program checkup, is fine. You can find a professional personal trainer by calling your local fitness center, looking in the phone book under "Personal Training," or asking friends for referrals. Look for a trainer who is certified by the National Strength and Conditioning Association (the top certification for personal trainers) or the American College of Sports Medicine (most often found working in hospital-based fitness centers).

> ### Suck It In
>
> Meet with a certified personal trainer every now and then who can help change your program for you, motivate you, and keep your successes coming.

Your Journey Toward Fitness

As a last word, remember that core fitness is all about making your body the best it can be for the long run. Never falter on the road to fitness: it's a long road that just keeps on going because fitness is more of a journey than a destination. We never really reach the end because there is always something more to achieve. So get to work and stay fit! I'll see you on that road.

The Least You Need to Know

◆ Core-conditioning results cannot always be seen, but they can be felt. Your motivation to continue challenging yourself has to come from the positive feeling of accomplishment you get, not from the mirror.

◆ Write down the details of each workout (exercises, sets, reps, and so on) so you have a record of what you have achieved and so you can remember where you have to go next.

◆ From time to time, hire a personal trainer to evaluate your program for you and provide some new ideas to keep you moving forward.

◆ When it comes to getting fit, it's more about the journey than the destination.

Glossary

abdominal cavity   The space between your lower ribs and the top of your pelvis, where most of your internal organs are located. This cavity is created by the abdominal muscles on the front and side, and the lower-back muscles and vertebrae in the back.

abdominals   Four muscles, including the rectus abdominis, internal and external obliques, and transversus abdominis, that help you bend forward, twist from side to side, and suck in your stomach.

aerobic endurance   The ability to maintain a given level of exercise intensity for a period of time, usually at least 20 minutes. Also called cardiovascular endurance.

aerobic training   A form of training that gets your heart rate up into your target zone and keeps it there for at least 20 minutes. Common methods include jogging, cycling, swimming, and skating.

asthma   A pulmonary disease characterized by a restricted airway and difficulty breathing.

balance   Being able to maintain a position without falling over, such as standing on one leg or sitting on top of a stability ball.

blood pressure   The pressure that blood exerts on the walls of your arteries every time your heart beats. Normal blood pressure is around 120/80. High blood pressure is anything over 140/90.

body sculpting   A type of exercise that focuses on developing your muscles into a particular shape using a combination of free weights, machines, and resistance-tubing exercises. The goal is to improve the way your body looks to you and others.

body weight   How much you weigh on the scales, usually measured in pounds. With regard to exercise, a "body weight" exercise uses only your weight for resistance.

cardiovascular exercise   Any exercise that increases your heart rate into your target zone and keeps it there for at least 20 minutes. Also called aerobic exercise.

cervical vertebrae   The seven vertebrae on the top of your spine, beginning at your skull and stopping just under your shoulders.

cool-down   The final part of your daily exercise program, in which you allow your heart rate to return to normal, you catch your breath, and you perform your flexibility training.

core conditioning   A type of exercise training that focuses on the deeper muscles of your torso, usually muscles you can't see. This training improves how you feel and how you move rather than how you look.

core temperature   The temperature inside any given muscle. A higher core temperature helps you move more easily and feel looser.

deep muscles   The muscles underneath the larger surface muscles. These muscles are usually much smaller and cannot be felt with your hands or seen in the mirror.

deep posterior muscles   The group of muscles that traverse the area from the bottom of your ribs to the top of your pelvis along your spine. These are also called the lower-back muscles.

energy systems   The body gets its energy from either aerobic or anaerobic processes. Whereas core conditioning relies on anaerobic (without oxygen) energy, cardiovascular training needs aerobic (with oxygen) energy. Anaerobic systems use mainly carbohydrates for fuel. Aerobic systems use more fats.

erector spinae   The illiocostalis, longissimus, and spinalis muscles of the lower back that work as a group to keep your spine erect, or straight.

estimated maximal heart rate   The fastest possible speed that your heart can beat, calculated as 220 minus your age.

exercise accumulation   The result of adding up smaller exercise sessions until you reach the total time you set as your goal.

extension   A movement characterized by a limb being straightened out or moved away from the core. Examples are when you stretch your leg away from your core or lift your arm over your head.

external oblique   One of the four abdominal muscles. Mainly responsible for rotating the trunk.

flexibility   The ability to move through a given range of motion without pain or stiffness. The more flexible your joints are, the easier it is to perform core-conditioning exercises.

flexion   A movement characterized by a limb being pulled in toward the core. An example is when you bend your knees toward your chest.

form   Proper execution of an exercise by following the steps exactly. Proper form helps prevent injury.

free weights   Exercise resistance in the form of steel or iron weights, such as barbells and dumbbells.

functional training   Another common term for core conditioning. "Functional" refers to how well the results of the exercise translate into daily life. A functional exercise is something that you can benefit from even when you aren't exercising.

glutes   A term for the three gluteus muscles: gluteus maximus, medius, and minimus. Also commonly called the butt muscles.

gluteus maximus   The largest of the glutes, responsible mainly for extension of the hip. This muscle is also a surface muscle that can be felt and seen in the mirror.

gluteus medius   The second layer of the glutes, just below the gluteus maximus. This muscle helps with rotation of the hip.

gluteus minimus   The smallest and deepest of the glute muscles. It also helps with hip rotation.

gravity   A source of resistance you can't escape unless you travel to outer space. The core muscles are always working against the force of gravity because gravity is always pushing you down toward the ground.

heart problems   Includes heart attacks, angina (chest pains), bypass surgery, and cardiovascular disease.

hip extension   The movement that occurs when you push your foot down toward the floor and away from your core.

hip flexion   The movement that occurs when you lift your foot and knee up toward your chest.

hyperextension   The movement that occurs when you lean backward from a standing position, as if you were looking at something on the ceiling or up in the air; you are bent over backward.

iliopsoas   A pair of muscles that are mainly responsible for flexion of the hip. Includes the iliacus and psoas major muscles.

illiocostalis   Part of the erector spinae group, this muscle helps keep the spine straight and assists in bending it to the side, when necessary.

intensity   How hard or difficult an exercise is. It can be measured in increased speed, more weight (a heavier medicine ball), or more time spent holding a position.

internal oblique   Part of the abdominal group, this muscle helps rotate the torso.

involuntary movements   Muscle actions that you don't control through conscious thought; they happen just because the brain knows they need to occur to help you move or stabilize another muscle.

lactic acid   A by-product of muscle contractions, this chemical builds up in the body and causes fatigue and possibly soreness.

lateral flexion   The movement that occurs when you bend or lean over to one side. The motion is possible because of the hip and vertebral joint's flexibility.

life schedule   All the things that take up your time during a normal day. This includes your work, play, family time, and hobbies.

localized blood flow   The amount of blood flow through a muscle being increased during exercise because the muscle needs more oxygen, which is delivered by the blood.

longissimus   A muscle that helps to extend the spine and neck from a bent-over position to a standing or straight position.

lumbar vertebrae   The five bottom vertebrae that form the base of your spine. These are the largest and strongest of all the vertebrae, but they also incur the most stress from normal movements.

maintenance   A type of training program in which you are not trying to make any improvements but are not losing any ground, either. You are keeping your fitness level exactly where it's at. Maintenance is fine for short periods, but you should always be striving for improvement.

medicine ball   A heavy ball that resembles a basketball, except that it weighs between 2 and 25 pounds.

metabolic disease   Includes diabetes mellitus, thyroid disorders, and renal or liver disease.

muscular endurance   The ability of a muscle to contract and move over and over again without getting tired.

pectineus   A muscle that both flexes and rotates the hip.

physical   An annual medical checkup done by your physician. A physical should include blood pressure measurement, body fat measurement, cholesterol check, heart rate measurement, and complete muscular and skeletal assessments.

Pilates   A form of exercise invented by Joseph Pilates that incorporates slow movements and lots of flexibility. This style of workout involves the use of special equipment made just for Pilates.

power   The ability to move quickly against a resistance, such as when you are performing a medicine ball wood chop.

principle of diminishing returns   More is not always better. This principle states that doing twice as much will not necessarily give you twice the results. The more you do, the smaller the return on your investment of time and energy becomes. During exercise, there is a point at which the body can do only so much before your form starts to go bad and the results drop off quickly.

principle of progression   If you want to see improvements, you have to work harder than you are used to. When you are able to do an exercise with ease, your body will not see any more results because it doesn't need to get any better. Progression means always working a little bit harder.

pulmonary disease   Includes chronic obstructive pulmonary disease, asthma, interstitial lung disease, and cystic fibrosis.

rectus abdominis   Part of the abdominal group, this is the biggest abdominal muscle on the surface. This muscle is commonly called the "six pack" because of the arrangement of the muscle fibers.

rectus femoris   A major hip flexor and part of the quadriceps thigh muscles.

repetitions   This term refers to how much of an exercise you perform. Each complete movement counts as one repetition.

resistance   Any force that acts to prevent you from moving. Resistance is everywhere in the form of gravity, and in the gym in the form of weights and machines.

resistance tubing   Normally made from very strong surgical-type tubing with handles at both ends, this form of resistance is infinitely adjustable because of the different sizes and lengths available. It's one of the most versatile methods of increasing your exercise intensity.

rest   The time between each exercise set or between each exercise. Rest can be either sitting still, walking, or performing an exercise for another muscle group.

rotation   Moving the body in the transverse plane, usually done by twisting at the hips and waist.

sartorius   A muscle that flexes the hip and rotates the torso.

sets   A group of repetitions done in a sequence. For example, one set may include 10 repetitions, and you may do three sets of that exercise.

spinalis   A muscle in the erector spinae group that helps to extend the vertebral column.

sports performance   How well you can perform a given sport, often determined by your level of conditioning.

stability ball   A large, very strong ball that is inflated and used in place of a chair or exercise bench. It produces an unstable surface upon which exercises are performed.

stabilizers   Muscles that contract and work to stabilize the spine, the arms or legs, or other muscles while a movement is being performed. Stabilizers don't actually produce the movement; they just brace the body.

strength   Typically measured by how much weight you can lift in a given exercise (such as the bench press). Within core conditioning, strength is measured by how well you can perform the exercise.

stretching   Extending a muscle from its normal resting length to a point at which you begin to feel the strain of the muscle "pulling" against the bones it's attached to.

surface muscles   The muscles on the "surface" of the body, just under the skin. Because of their size, these muscles often hide the deep muscles.

target heart rate   This is the heart rate range in which you should perform your core cardiovascular training.

tensor fasciae latae   A muscle that flexes the hip.

thoracic vertebrae   A group of 12 bones located between the cervical and lumbar vertebrae. They are found in the middle of your back.

three-dimensional movement   Any motion that includes a combination of any three of the following actions: flexion, lateral flexion, hyperextension, and rotation.

transversus abdominis   A member of the abdominal group. This muscle is mainly responsible for pulling the abdominal cavity in toward the spine (such as when you suck in your stomach).

vertebrae   Each one of the stack of 24 bones that make up your spine.

voluntary movements   Actions that you decide to make and have conscious control of (such as when you decide to turn this page).

weight machines   Exercise equipment used in body-sculpting and weight-training programs. They involve stacks of weights connected to cables and pulleys. Each machine normally works only one or two muscles in a particular fashion.

weight training   A type of exercise that focuses on increasing your muscular strength and size.

yoga   A type of exercise that focuses on slow movements that improve your flexibility.

Equipment and Training Resources

When it's time to pick up some new core-conditioning equipment, think long-term. You don't want to purchase something that will wear out in a few weeks, so try and stay away from department store equipment. The companies listed here are suppliers to the major health club chains, professional sports teams, and personal trainers. They have the good stuff that will take a beating and is built to last. Sure, you'll pay a few extra dollars, but it's better than having to buy the lower-quality stuff over and over again.

If you decide it's time to get some professional advice on how these exercises can be suited just for you, then it's time to find a personal trainer. If you type the term "personal trainer" into an Internet search engine, you will get millions of hits. To narrow this down, I've included the organizations that have the best educated trainers on their roles. These aren't fly-by-night groups. You can bet that if a trainer's name is on their referral list, they know what they are talking about, and can assist you in getting the most from this book.

Resistance Tubing, Medicine Balls, Stability Balls, and Other Equipment

Champion Sports
PO Box 368
Marlboro, NJ 07746
1-888-980-1200
www.championsports.com

Fitness First
PO Box 251
Shawnee Mission, KS 66201
1-800-421-1791
www.fitness1st.com

Fitness Wholesale
895-A Hampshire Road
Stow, OH 44224
1-800-537-5512
www.fwonline.com

M-F Athletic/Perform Better
11 Amflex Drive
Cranston, RI 02920
1-800-682-6950
www.performbetter.com

Power Systems
PO Box 31709
Knoxville, TN 37930
1-800-321-6975
www.power-systems.com

Sportsmith
5925 S. 118th East Avenue
Tulsa, OK 74146
1-800-713-2880
www.sportsmith.net

SPRI Products, Inc.
1600 Northwind Blvd.
Libertyville, IL 60048
1-800-222-7774
www.spriproducts.com

Personal Trainers

American College of Sports Medicine
PO Box 1440
Indianapolis, IN 46206
1-800-486-5643
www.acsm.org

IDEA Health and Fitness Association
10455 Pacific Center Ct.
San Diego, CA 92121
1-800-999-IDEA
www.ideafit.com

National Strength and Conditioning Association
1885 Bob Johnson Drive
Colorado Springs, CO 80906
1-800-815-6826
www.nsca-lift.org

Sample Workout Plans and Log

Beginner Workouts

These workouts are for those of you who are new to core conditioning and want to get started without getting too sore. Start with no more than three workouts each week, with at least a day of rest between each workout. Each workout can be completed all at one time or can be split up into several smaller workouts. Be sure to do the exercises in the order listed.

Body Weight Workout

1. Abdominal crunch: 2 sets of 15–20 reps
2. Oblique crunch: 2 sets of 15–20 reps per side
3. Wall roll-up: 2 sets of 10 reps
4. Pointer: 2 sets of 5 reps; hold each rep 15 seconds
5. Bridging: 1 set of 10 reps; hold each rep 10 seconds

Resistance Tubing Workout

1. Twisting punch: 2 sets of 10–15 reps per side
2. Overhead crunch: 3 sets of 30 reps
3. Two-hand twist: 2 sets of 10–15 reps

Medicine Ball Workout

1. Wood chop: 2 sets of 10 reps
2. Crunch twist: 2 sets of 15 reps per side
3. Overhead balance: 2 sets of 15 seconds per side
4. Prone back extension: 3 sets of 20 seconds

Stability Ball Workout

1. Ball crunch: 2 sets of 15 reps
2. Glute ham raise: 2 sets of 10 reps
3. Ball bridging: 3 sets of 30 seconds each
4. Inclined Superman: 2 sets of 30 seconds each
5. Kneeling tuck: 2 sets of 10 reps

Advanced Workouts

These workouts should be attempted only after you have completed all the beginning exercises and workouts. They are a little more intense and a bit longer, so plan your workout time accordingly and work your way up to three or four workouts a week.

Advanced Body Weight Workout

1. Cycling: 2 sets of 60 seconds each direction
2. Balanced toe touch: 3 sets of 20 reps each side
3. Double crunch: 2 sets of 40 reps
4. Tuck: 3 sets of 20 reps
5. Modified bridging: 2 sets of 60 seconds on each side
6. Windmill: 4 sets of 10 reps each side

Advanced Resistance Tubing Workout

1. Diagonal wood chop: 3 sets of 10 reps each side
2. Balanced side pull: 2 sets of 12 reps each side
3. One-arm throw: 2 sets of 10 reps each side
4. Granny pass: 3 sets of 10 reps
5. Lying tuck: 3 sets of 15 reps
6. Seated Russian twist: 3 sets of 10 reps

Advanced Medicine Ball Workout

1. Walking Russian twist: 3 sets of 30 steps
2. Rocky abs: 3 sets of 60 seconds
3. Pendulum: 3 sets of 20 reps
4. Diagonal throw: 2 sets of 10 throws each side
5. Overhead throw: 3 sets of 15 reps

Advanced Stability Ball Workout

1. Back bridge: 2 sets of 60 seconds
2. Walkout: 3 sets of 10 reps
3. Glute lift: 3 sets of 15 reps
4. Leg twist: 3 sets of 30 reps
5. Moguls: 2 sets of 15 reps
6. Double balance: 2 sets of 60 seconds

Sample Workout Log

You can design your workout log any way you like. Some people like to use spiral notebooks; others keep track on their computers. Whichever method you choose, the important components are a list of the exercises you do, how many reps and sets of each exercise you complete, how much rest you take between sets, the total time of your workout (so you can see how long it takes you and how your speed improves), and a space for comments on how your workout felt. Here's an example layout:

Date: Tuesday 8/15/05

Exercise	Sets/Reps	Rest Between Sets
Walking Russian twist	3 sets of 25 steps	30 seconds
Rocky abs	3 sets of 60 seconds (Note: 40 reps first set, 38 reps second set, 35 reps third set)	30 seconds
Pendulum	3 sets of 20 reps	15 seconds
Diagonal throw	2 sets of 12 reps/side	30 seconds
Overhead throw	3 sets of 15 reps	45 seconds

Total workout time: 38 minutes

Comments: Hard workout today, felt strong and energized starting out, got winded after rocky abs, took 3 minutes rest between each exercise today. Very tired at the end, drank some water, rested about 10 minutes, ready to go. Can't wait until tomorrow's workout!!

Index

O